Median Arcuate Ligament Syndrome

Daniel Shouhed • Omar M. Ghanem
Kevin El-Hayek
Editors

Median Arcuate Ligament Syndrome

State of the Art Management

Springer

Editors
Daniel Shouhed
Robotic Surgical Institute of Southern California
Beverly Hills, CA, USA

Omar M. Ghanem
Department of Surgery
Mayo Clinic
Rochester, MN, USA

Kevin El-Hayek
Department of Surgery
The MetroHealth System, Case Western Reserve University School of Medicine
Cleveland, OH, USA

ISBN 978-3-031-80742-8 ISBN 978-3-031-80740-4 (eBook)
https://doi.org/10.1007/978-3-031-80740-4

This Springer imprint is published by the registered company Springer Nature Switzerland AG
The registered company address is: Gewerbestrasse 11, 6330 Cham, Switzerland

To my parents, Johnny and Shideh, for their unconditional love and support. To my children, Remi, Julian and Dylan, for giving me new purpose in life. Most importantly, to my loving wife, Amy, who always believed in me and convinced me that it is possible to specialize in a disease process as rare as MALS.

Daniel Shouhed

To my wife, Nadine, whose continual encouragement and unwavering support are the foundation of my success as a father and as a surgeon. To my daughter Yvanna and my son Yuri whose love inspires me every single day. To my parents and family and their sacrifices for me to be where I am now. To my forever mentor, Dr. Michael Kendrick, who taught me and still guides me in my surgical career.

Omar M. Ghanem

To my mentors in minimally invasive surgery, Bipan Chand and Matthew Kroh. I am truly grateful for the foundation you provided to me in endoscopic, laparoscopic, and robotic surgery. Not only did you transfer technical skills, but more importantly you helped me develop the harder skill of surgical judgement. To Matt, you introduced me to MALS when I was still a trainee, and the complexity of the disease inspired me to pursue a deeper understanding of it. In large part, that pursuit has culminated with this textbook, which I am certain will improve the understanding of MALS for medical, surgical, and patient communities.

Kevin El-Hayek

Preface

Despite being identified as a pathologic human condition over a century ago, median arcuate ligament syndrome (MALS) continues to be a controversial diagnosis for many in the medical field. That said, MALS has emerged as a significant clinical condition, attracting attention from healthcare professionals and researchers worldwide. Characterized by the compression of the celiac artery and surrounding neural structures by the median arcuate ligament, MALS presents a complex and multifaceted challenge in both diagnosis and management. The intricacies of this syndrome, from its diverse symptoms to the variety of treatment modalities available, necessitate a comprehensive, in-depth exploration.

Median Arcuate Ligament Syndrome: State of the Art Management is a seminal textbook that brings together the collective expertise of leading authorities in the field from around the globe. This book is meticulously designed to serve as the definitive guide for healthcare professionals, offering an exhaustive overview of MALS, its pathophysiology, diagnostic processes, and treatment options.

This textbook begins with an exploration of the historical context of MALS, tracing the evolution of understanding and treatment of this condition. Understanding the pathophysiology of MALS is crucial, as it lays the groundwork for comprehending the subsequent chapters on anatomy, including normal anatomical variations and their implications for MALS.

A thorough discussion on the symptoms, presentation, and differential diagnosis of MALS is then provided, helping clinicians recognize and distinguish it from other conditions with similar presentations. The diagnostic arsenal for MALS is vast, encompassing duplex ultrasound, CT angiogram, visceral angiography, and celiac plexus block, all of which are discussed in detail to aid in accurate and timely diagnosis.

A unique aspect of this textbook is its comprehensive coverage of conditions associated with MALS. The conditions include postural orthostatic tachycardia syndrome (POTS), Ehlers–Danlos syndrome (EDS), gastroparesis, mast cell activation syndrome (MCAS), nutcracker syndrome, May–Thurner syndrome, pelvic congestion syndrome, and superior mesenteric artery syndrome (SMAS). These chapters underscore the interconnected nature of these conditions and their relevance in the context of MALS.

Next, treatment strategies are extensively covered, with dedicated chapters on nonoperative management and various surgical approaches, including open, laparoscopic, and robotic techniques. Special attention is given to perioperative anesthesia considerations and the specific challenges of managing MALS in pediatric patients. This book also addresses potential complications of MALS surgery and long-term outcomes, including the possibility of recurrent MALS.

Finally, recognizing the critical role of patient advocacy and the value of online support groups, this textbook concludes with a chapter that highlights the importance of these resources in the journey of MALS patients. We believe this is one of the first examples of including the patient's voice—the most important yet often overlooked voice—in a surgical textbook.

Median Arcuate Ligament Syndrome: State of the Art Management stands as a testament to the global collaboration of experts committed to advancing the understanding and treatment of MALS. It is an invaluable resource for surgeons, gastroenterologists, radiologists, anesthesiologists, and all healthcare professionals involved in the care of patients with MALS.

Beverly Hills, CA, USA — Daniel Shouhed
Rochester, MN, USA — Omar M. Ghanem
Cleveland, OH, USA — Kevin El-Hayek

Acknowledgements

As editors-in-chief, we would like to acknowledge our co-editor, Dr. Omar Ghanem. Your input in shaping this textbook has improved the scientific merit exponentially. It was truly a pleasure embarking on this journey with you, and we look forward to future collaborations to advance our understanding of this complex disorder. We would also like to offer our gratitude to all the authors who contributed to this important textbook. Finally, to the primary inspiration to take on this project—our patients. Your stories inspire us to keep finding better ways to treat you. We are grateful that you have placed your trust in us.

Daniel Shouhed and Kevin El-Hayek

Contents

Contributors

Benjamin Abraham Department of Anesthesiology and Pain Management, Cleveland Clinic, Cleveland, OH, USA

Imad Absah Division of Pediatric Gastroenterology and Hepatology, Mayo Clinic, Rochester, MN, USA

Nicolas M. Mas D. Alessandro Department of Anesthesiology and Pain Management, The MetroHealth System, Case Western Reserve University School of Medicine, Cleveland, OH, USA

Michael M. Awad Department of Surgery, Section of Minimally Invasive Surgery, School of Medicine, Washington University, St. Louis, MO, USA

Juan S. Barajas-Gamboa Cleveland Clinic Abu Dhabi, Abu Dhabi, UAE

Jonathan C. Bartko, MD Harrington Heart and Vascular Institute, University Hospitals, Cleveland, OH, USA

Case Western Reserve University School of Medicine, Cleveland, OH, USA

Amanda Belluzzi Department of General Surgery, Rovigo Hospital, Rovigo, Italy

Department of Metabolic and Abdominal Wall Reconstructive Surgery, Mayo Clinic, Rochester, MN, USA

Natalie Chao School of Medicine, University of Maryland, Baltimore, MD, USA

Jennifer Curti Division of General Surgery, Intermountain Medical Group, Intermountain Health, LDS Hospital, Salt Lake City, UT, USA

Jamie DeCicco Cleveland Clinic Lerner College of Medicine of Case Western Reserve University, Cleveland, OH, USA

Division of General Surgery, Department of Surgery, The MetroHealth System, Cleveland, OH, USA

Vipul Dhumak Department of Anesthesiology and Pain Management, The MetroHealth System, Case Western Reserve University School of Medicine, Cleveland, OH, USA

Eleanor Dunlap Division of Vascular Surgery, University of Maryland Medical Center, Baltimore, MD, USA

Division of Vascular Surgery, Department of Surgery, University of Maryland, Baltimore, MD, USA

Eric Dutson Department of Surgery, Huggins Hospital, Wolfeboro, NH, USA

Kevin El-Hayek Department of Surgery, The MetroHealth System, Case Western Reserve University School of Medicine, Cleveland, OH, USA

Katherine Fay School of Medicine, Emory University, Atlanta, GA, USA

William D. Gerull Department of Surgery, Section of Minimally Invasive Surgery, School of Medicine, Washington University, St. Louis, MO, USA

Omar M. Ghanem Department of Surgery, Mayo Clinic, Rochester, MN, USA

Diane Gilmore National MALS Foundation, Dedham, MA, USA

Laura Gilmore National MALS Foundation, Dedham, MA, USA

Clement Ho Department of Anesthesiology and Pain Management, Cleveland Clinic, Cleveland, OH, USA

Tanya M. Holton National MALS Foundation, Dedham, MA, USA

Jessica Johnson Cleveland Clinic Lerner College of Medicine of Case Western Reserve University, Cleveland, OH, USA

Manju Kalra Division of Vascular and Endovascular Surgery, Mayo Clinic, Rochester, MN, USA

Peter Kanuika Department of Surgery, The MetroHealth System, Cleveland, OH, USA

Matthew Kroh Cleveland Clinic Lerner College of Medicine of Case Western Reserve University, Digestive Disease Institute, Cleveland Clinic, Cleveland, OH, USA

Gabriela Lozano Robotic Surgical Institute of Southern California, Beverly Hills, CA, USA

Kamal Abi Mosleh Department of Metabolic and Abdominal Wall Reconstructive Surgery, Mayo Clinic, Rochester, MN, USA

Khanjan H. Nagarsheth School of Medicine, University of Maryland, Baltimore, MD, USA

Division of Vascular Surgery, University of Maryland Medical Center, Baltimore, MD, USA

Woosup Michael Park, MD Harrington Heart and Vascular Institute, University Hospitals, Cleveland, OH, USA

Case Western Reserve University School of Medicine, Cleveland, OH, USA

Ankit D. Patel School of Medicine, Emory University, Atlanta, GA, USA

Suzanne Keppley Peek National MALS Foundation, Dedham, MA, USA

Joshua Plant Division of Vascular Surgery, University of Maryland Medical Center, Baltimore, MD, USA

Michael Platten Department of Anesthesiology and Pain Management, The MetroHealth System, Case Western Reserve University School of Medicine, Cleveland, OH, USA

Todd E. Rasmussen Department of Vascular Surgery, Mayo Clinic, Rochester, MN, USA

Nathan G. Richards Department of Surgery, University of Utah, Salt Lake City, UT, USA

Division of General Surgery, Intermountain Medical Group, Intermountain Health, LDS Hospital, Salt Lake City, UT, USA

Gustavo Romero-Velez Cleveland Clinic, Cleveland, OH, USA

Aida K. Sarcon Department of Surgery, Mayo Clinic, Rochester, MN, USA

Melinda S. Schaller Division of Vascular and Endovascular Surgery, Mayo Clinic, Rochester, MN, USA

Robin Insley Schrader National MALS Foundation, Dedham, MA, USA

Daniel Shouhed Robotic Surgical Institute of Southern California, Beverly Hills, CA, USA

Maninder Singh Department of Anesthesiology and Pain Management, The MetroHealth System, Case Western Reserve University School of Medicine, Cleveland, OH, USA

Leif Sorensen Department of Surgery, University of Utah, Salt Lake City, UT, USA

Krysta M. Sutyak Department of Surgery, University of Nebraska Medical Center, Omaha, NE, USA

Department of Surgery, Children's Nebraska, Omaha, NE, USA

Luis Tollinche Department of Anesthesiology and Pain Management, The MetroHealth System, Case Western Reserve University School of Medicine, Cleveland, OH, USA

Robert Wilson Cleveland Clinic Lerner College of Medicine of Case Western Reserve University, Cleveland, OH, USA

Department of Neurology, Neuromuscular Center, Cleveland Clinic, Cleveland, OH, USA

Abdalla E. Zarroug Department of Surgery, University of Nebraska Medical Center, Omaha, NE, USA

Department of Surgery, Children's Nebraska, Omaha, NE, USA

Chapter 1
The History and Evolution of Treatment Modalities for Median Arcuate Ligament Syndrome

Nathan G. Richards, Leif Sorensen, Eric Dutson, and Daniel Shouhed

Introduction

The first description of median arcuate ligament syndrome (MALS) dates all the way back to 1917. It wasn't until nearly half a century later that the first patient was treated for MALS. There has been a major evolution in the diagnosis and treatment of this rare disorder. Like many other procedures, surgeons have adopted a minimally invasive approach over the last 20 years. A better understanding of the pathophysiology of MALS as well as the adoption of a minimally invasive approach has drastically increased the recognition and treatment of this debilitating disorder. This chapter aims to explore the historical progression of treatment modalities for MALS, highlighting key milestones and contemporary approaches.

N. G. Richards (✉)
Department of Surgery, University of Utah, Salt Lake City, UT, USA

Division of General Surgery, Intermountain Medical Group, Intermountain Health, LDS Hospital, Salt Lake City, UT, USA
e-mail: Nathan.richards@imail.org

L. Sorensen
Department of Surgery, University of Utah, Salt Lake City, UT, USA

E. Dutson
Department of Surgery, Huggins Hospital, Wolfeboro, NH, USA

D. Shouhed
Robotic Surgical Institute of Southern California, Beverly Hills, CA, USA

D. Shouhed et al. (eds.), *Median Arcuate Ligament Syndrome*,
https://doi.org/10.1007/978-3-031-80740-4_1

History: Etiology

In 1963, PT Harjola first described what he termed celiac artery compression syndrome. In that paper, Dr. Harjola records the clinical presentation, diagnosis, and surgical treatment of a 57-year-old male whose presenting symptoms included postprandial epigastric pain and nausea. Visceral and aortic angiography demonstrated near-occlusion of the celiac artery with exhalation, a finding never before noted in his practice or the literature. Dr. Harjola hypothesized that an external structure, the median arcuate ligament rising off the diaphragm, was compressing the origin of the celiac artery at the aorta. By cutting that ligament, Harjola conjectured that he could release the compression, leading to an improvement in symptoms and the patient's quality of life. He performed a laparotomy and dissected the right crus of the diaphragm. He identified the median arcuate ligament and divided it, releasing an obvious stenosis of the celiac artery. The patient's symptoms improved significantly. In his initial case report, Dr. Harjola coined the term "celiac artery compression syndrome" [1].

Nearly 2 years later, in 1965, Dr. Dunbar's seminal work reinforced Dr. Harjola's findings as he published his initial case series of 15 patients who also presented with postprandial epigastric pain, weight loss, and nausea. Thirteen of the 15 patients improved after the division of the median arcuate ligament and the resultant decompression of the celiac artery [2]. In further work to establish the diagnosis, in a 1968 article entitled "Celiac Axis Syndrome: abdominal angina caused by external compression of the celiac artery," Dr. Harjola records a series of 13 patients on whom he had performed decompressive release. Nine of his thirteen patients "became asymptomatic, three had mild epigastric pain, and one failed to improve after dissection of the constricting tissue." Interestingly, Dr. Harjola describes the stenosis as caused by either "the margin of the aortic hiatus pressing the celiac axis against the aorta [,] by the fibrotic celiac ganglion constricting the celiac artery in a ringlike manner, or by a combination of both" [3]. Dr. Charles Rob, in 1967, described "a previously undefined cause of symptomatic celiac artery stenosis, one of external compression of the origin of the celiac artery by the surrounding fibrous and neural tissue of the celiac ganglion" [4]. In 1972, Martinez et al. published an appropriately titled article that captured a review of the then-current literature and the prevailing sentiment around MALS that would persist for several decades. Their paper was called "The Relentless Symptom Complex of Undiagnosed Celiac Artery Compression" [5].

For these vascular pioneers and others not cited here, the predominant hypothesis of the etiology of MALS clearly focused on intestinal ischemia secondary to celiac artery compression. Regardless of what is causing the compression, a stenosed celiac artery origin is the culprit for the relentless symptom complex. The theory, essentially gastric claudication, posits that the increased oxygen and glucose needs of the contracting, activated stomach are unmet due to blood flow restriction at the origin of the celiac artery by the median arcuate ligament. Interestingly, despite Dr. Rob and Dr. Harjola both having identified fibrotic, rigid ganglionic tissue as a potential cause of the stenosis, it does not appear that a neurogenic etiology was considered at the time. In fact, for the next 50 years, the predominant thrust in diagnosing and treating MALS focused on restoring blood flow to the stomach.

Unfortunately, controversy dogged MALS as a legitimate diagnosis over this same time period. This controversy largely resulted from less-than-stellar improvement after surgery, a paucity of evidence confirming gastric claudication, including the unreliability and inconsistency of gastric exercise tonometry, and variation in surgical approach and technique to obtain results. In most cases, patients with an appropriate history of symptoms, including postprandial epigastric pain, persistent nausea, weight loss, and other GI disturbances, would be subjected to confirmatory tests. These tests often include but are not limited to selected visceral arteriography, CT angiography, MR angiography, Doppler ultrasound of the celiac artery, etc. These tests, if confirmatory, would elicit a patient journey to the operating room for an attempted decompression or revascularization. Outcomes were mixed, and durable success was difficult to predict. This conundrum is highlighted in the title of a 2007 article written by Drs. Gloviczki and Duncan, "Treatment of celiac artery compression syndrome: does it really exist?" [6].

As early as 2012, many MALS practitioners started to wonder if it was time to reconsider the long-held hypothesis of intestinal or gastric ischemia secondary to vascular insufficiency. The celiac plexus, a network of autonomic nerves located in close proximity to the celiac artery, has emerged as a likely contributor to the pathogenesis of MALS. Compression of the celiac artery by the median arcuate ligament may lead to secondary irritation or compression of the celiac plexus, resulting in visceral hypersensitivity and neuropathic pain. This theory has gained traction in recent years, offering new insights into the diverse clinical manifestations of MALS beyond arterial insufficiency alone. One major problem with arterial insufficiency (and resultant visceral angina) being the dominant cause of symptomatology is basic anatomy. Though there seems to be a bimodal age distribution for patients diagnosed with MALS, the typical patient is a young, slender woman in whom it can be safely assumed that no advanced atherosclerotic disease is present. As this is surely the case with all such young patients, even a total occlusion of the celiac artery would not cause visceral ischemia due to retrograde flow from the superior mesenteric artery (SMA) through the pancreatic arcades. This has, in fact, been shown on duplex ultrasonography and angiography in patients with severe compression of the celiac trunk [7, 8]. Nevertheless, such an occlusion by external compression of a healthy artery could cause a local inflammatory response, which is often seen intraoperatively during MALR. This inflammatory process can itself cause irritation of the celiac ganglia.

Treating teams turned to celiac plexus blocks with more regularity and found an advantage in their predictability of postsurgical clinical response. In 2014, Brody et al. [7] declared in print that MALS was likely neurogenic instead of vascular as a primary pathology. Several other papers emerged, echoing this declaration, including Weber et al. and Kim et al. in 2016 [8, 9]. By 2022, Barbon et al. boldly stated that "Clinical response to celiac plexus block confirms the neurogenic etiology of median arcuate ligament syndrome" in the Journal of Vascular and Interventional Radiology. They describe a single-institution, retrospective cohort study of 96 clinically diagnosed patients with MALS. CT-guided percutaneous celiac plexus blocks were performed 103 times in this cohort. Eighty percent of these patients had postprandial pain score decrease from an average score of 6.3 to 0.9 ($p < 0.001$). Postprandial nausea decreased from 37.9% to 11.6% ($P < 0.001$). Importantly, the authors note that "pain relief did not correlate with the presence of celiac arterial abnormalities" on preop imaging. "This supports neuropathy as the primary etiology of MALS and suggests that the absence of celiac stenosis should not be used as an exclusion criterion" [10]. These data support a neurogenic etiology of MALS and underscore necessary changes in surgical technique to incorporate celiac ganglionectomy and neurolysis as primary components of MALR instead of just a division of the median arcuate ligament.

History: Treatment

The surgical treatment of MALS has evolved with time and an increasing understanding of its etiology. In the 1960s through the mid-1990s, MALS surgery was exclusively done via an upper midline laparotomy incision. The principles of this surgical approach include obtaining vascular control of the celiac artery and branches, dissection of the median arcuate ligament and the involved celiac ganglion, and division of any compressing fibers. The late 1980s saw the explosion of laparoscopic surgery, which revolutionized patient outcomes despite challenges in dealing with the increased learning curve for surgeons. The use of minimally invasive surgical techniques continued to expand through the 1990s and included transitioning MALR from open to laparoscopic [11, 12].

With building expertise in laparoscopic surgery, there was a definite shift toward minimally invasive surgery as a preferred approach to dealing with MALS, and FDA approval of surgical robotic systems in the early 2000s added another way to approach this technically difficult operation. A growing interest in and recognition of MALS, along with improved technical experience and equipment, led to a surge of publications related to MALS. As the presence of surgical robotic systems continued to expand, there has been at least one publication showing a 50% reduction in operative times when using a robotic approach to surgery versus a laparoscopic approach [13].

In recent years, endovascular approaches have emerged as promising alternatives to traditional open surgery for various vascular surgical pathologies, including MALS. Endovascular interventions, including angioplasty and stenting of the celiac artery, offer a less invasive option with reduced morbidity and faster recovery times. However, endovascular techniques' long-term durability and efficacy remain areas of ongoing research and debate. Additionally, if the cause of symptoms is neuropathic and not ischemia, endovascular angioplasty and/or stenting is likely to exacerbate an already existing nerve compression. Given the convincing support for a neurogenic basis of MALS, the efficacy of endovascular intervention to treat a syndrome that may not be vascular in nature is controversial.

Conclusion

Recognizing the complex etiology and varied clinical manifestations of MALS, a multidisciplinary approach involving gastroenterologists, gastrointestinal surgeons, vascular surgeons, and interventional radiologists has become increasingly important. Patient selection is key to assuring appropriate symptomatic and patient safety outcomes. As our understanding of MALS continues to evolve, future research directions aim to elucidate the underlying pathophysiology and identify novel therapeutic targets. Advances in minimally invasive techniques, personalized medicine, and collaborative research efforts hold the potential to further improve outcomes and quality of life for patients with MALS.

References

1. Dunbar JD, et al. Compression of the celiac trunk and abdominal angina: preliminary report of 15 cases. Am J Roentgenol. 1965;95(3):731–44.
2. Duffy AJ, et al. Management of median arcuate ligament syndrome: a new paradigm. Ann Vasc Surg. 2009;23(6):778–84.
3. Harjola P-T, Lahtiharju A. Celiac axis syndrome: abdominal angina caused by external compression of the celiac artery. Am J Surg. 1968;115(6):864–9.
4. Snyder MA, Mahoney EB, Rob CG. Symptomatic celiac artery stenosis due to constriction by the neurofibrous tissue of the celiac ganglion. Surgery. 1967;61(3):372–6.
5. Martinez NS, Khan AH. The relentless symptom complex of undiagnosed celiac artery compression. Angiology. 1972;23(4):198–204.
6. Gloviczki P, Duncan AA. Treatment of celiac artery compression syndrome: does it really exist? Perspect Vasc Surg Endovasc Ther. 2007;19(3):259–63.
7. Bowersox JC, et al. Duplex ultrasonography in the diagnosis of celiac and mesenteric artery occlusive disease. J Vasc Surg. 1991;14(6):780–8.
8. Rizzo A, et al. Celiac artery occlusion from median arcuate ligament compression complicating a hemorrhagic duodenal ulcer repair. J Vasc Surg Cases Innov Tech. 2024;10(1):101371.
9. Brody F, Richards NG. Median arcuate ligament release. J Am Coll Surg. 2014;219(4):e45–50.
10. Weber JM, et al. Median arcuate ligament syndrome is not a vascular disease. Ann Vasc Surg. 2016;30:22–7.
11. Kim EN, et al. Median arcuate ligament syndrome—review of this rare disease. JAMA Surg. 2016;151(5):471–7.
12. Barbon DA, et al. Clinical response to celiac plexus block confirms the neurogenic etiology of median arcuate ligament syndrome. J Vasc Interv Radiol. 2021;32(7):1081–7.
13. Dordoni L, et al. Celiac artery compression syndrome: successful laparoscopic treatment - a case report. Vasc Endovasc Surg. 2002;36(4):317–21.
14. Roseborough GS. Laparoscopic management of celiac artery compression syndrome. J Vasc Surg. 2009;50(1):124–33.
15. Khrucharoen U, et al. Short- and intermediate-term clinical outcome comparison between laparoscopic and robotic-assisted median arcuate ligament release. J Robot Surg. 2020;14(1):123–9.

Chapter 2
Pathophysiology of Median Arcuate Ligament Syndrome

William D. Gerull and Michael M. Awad

Introduction

The pathophysiology of median arcuate ligament syndrome (MALS) remains poorly understood. Several hypotheses have been proposed focusing on vasculogenic and neurogenic etiologies. Here, we discuss the relevant anatomy of the celiac trunk and surrounding structures and then detail the proposed causes of MALS.

Anatomy

The MAL is a diaphragmatic structure of arch-like fascia linking the right and left diaphragmatic crura. The diaphragmatic crura typically originate from the anterior aspect of the L1–L4 vertebral bodies. In this region, the MAL forms the anterior-most aspect of the aortic hiatus and permits passage of the abdominal aorta through the diaphragm. The aortic hiatus is most commonly found at T12-L1 of the vertebral column.

Traveling caudally on the aorta, the celiac artery (CA), superior mesenteric artery (SMA), and inferior mesenteric artery (IMA) originate from the anterior abdominal aorta. These structures have the most common vertebral positions of T12 for the CA, L1 for the SMA, L3 for the IMA [1]. The CA origin may vary anywhere from T11-L1 [2].

W. D. Gerull (✉) · M. M. Awad
Department of Surgery, Section of Minimally Invasive Surgery, School of Medicine, Washington University, St. Louis, MO, USA
e-mail: wgerull@wustl.edu; awadm@wustl.edu

D. Shouhed et al. (eds.), *Median Arcuate Ligament Syndrome*,
https://doi.org/10.1007/978-3-031-80740-4_2

The celiac ganglia are positioned on the anterolateral sides of the CA trunk. These are the largest sympathetic ganglia in the body, connected by the celiac plexus [1]. They provide sympathetic innervation signals to, and transmit visceral pain signals from, the foregut organs. The left ganglion is often a single mass, while the right ganglion is a complex of one to seven smaller interconnected ganglion masses with large rope-like cords [3]. The celiac plexus connects these ganglia and forms a dense network of nerve bundles traveling superiorly and inferiorly around the CA.

Vasculogenic Theory: Compression of the Celiac Artery

MALS is thought to involve external mechanical compression of the celiac artery by the MAL [4]. There are multiple components of CA compression, both temporal and anatomical.

The MAL is in close proximity to the CA and may overlap the CA and cause impingement. The most common CA anatomy includes a trifurcation into the splenic, left gastric, and common hepatic arteries. There is a great deal of anatomic variation in the gastric blood supply, and each of these arteries directly or indirectly supplies the stomach—the splenic artery through the short gastrics, the common hepatic artery through the right gastric, right and left gastroepiploic arteries, and the left gastric artery directly (Fig. 2.1). Immediately after eating, the stomach recruits more blood flow. This may explain the epigastric location of symptoms experienced immediately after eating regardless of the type of food. In addition, compression of

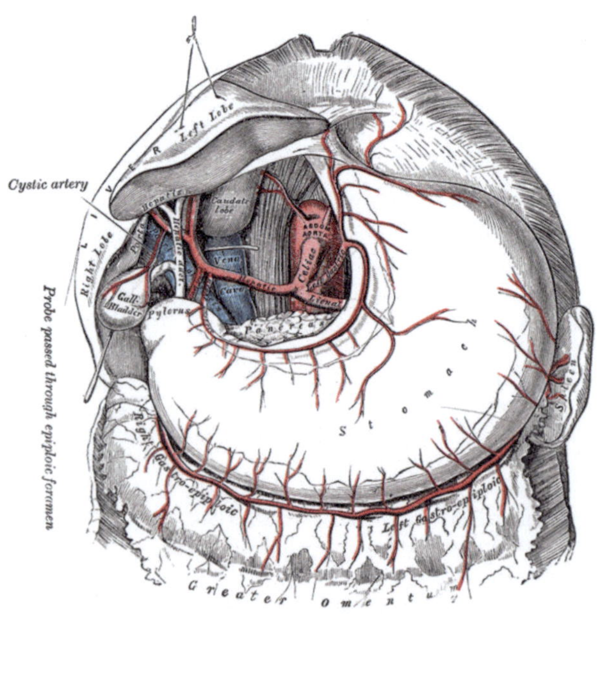

Fig. 2.1 Celiac artery anatomy. Case courtesy of Donna D'Souza, Radiopaedia.org, rID: 36176

the CA is commonly due to a more caudal location of the MAL rather than the more typical cranial origin of the CA [3]. Up to 33% of the general population may have a degree of CA compression as seen on routine imaging and cadaveric dissection [5, 6]. However, a much smaller percentage experience symptoms from CA compression and clinically develop MALS. There is a great deal of anatomic variation in the gastric blood supply. The difference in collateral and redundant blood supply, in combination with CA compression, may explain why some individuals are more or less symptomatic.

Specifically examining the anatomic importance of the CA origin in MALS pathology, in a study of 36 cadaveric specimens, Dyches et al. found that an acute angle of the CA origin was correlated with increased MAL/CA overlap. This suggests that the overlap of the MAL onto the CA most likely causes an acute angle of the CA rather than an inherently acute angle of the CA origin. In addition, they found no correlation between the vertebral height of the CA and the observed MAL/CA overlap. This suggests that individuals with MALS are more likely to have an inferiorly positioned or elongated diaphragm rather than a high CA origin [6].

Importantly, the compression of the CA may be exacerbated during the respiratory cycle. During expiration, the diaphragm rises causing the free edge of the MAL to pull up on the CA/aorta junction, causing a "hooking" effect on the celiac artery [7] (Fig. 2.2). This can be seen in dynamic cross-sectional imaging or angiography. This respiratory variation can significantly affect flow through the CA by 50–100% in some cases. Knowledge of this respiratory variation on CA blood flow can be used in the diagnostic workup of MALS, discussed further in other chapters.

An additional vasculogenic theory details a steal syndrome related to CA stenosis causing midgut ischemia. Importantly, the chronic compression of the CA can lead to the development of collateral blood flow, which often prevents the true development of ischemia [8]. This theory suggests that in a postprandial state, the SMA diverts blood flow to these large collateral vessels to supply the diminutive

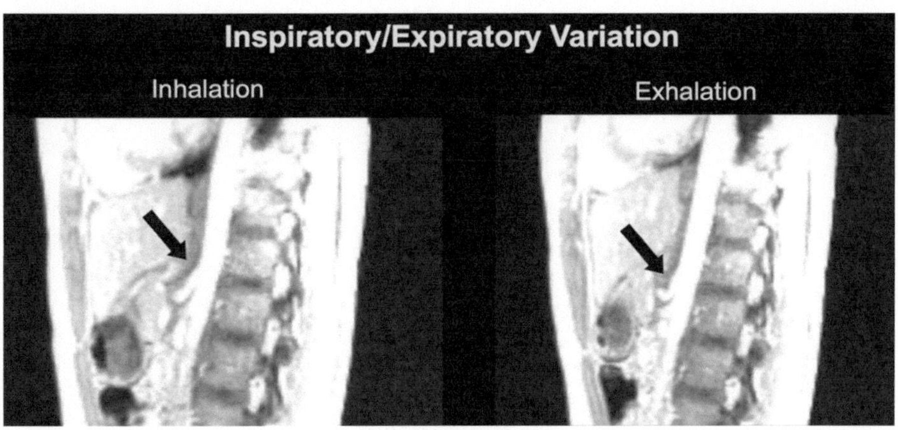

Fig. 2.2 Computer tomography imaging of the inspiratory and expiratory variation with the "hooking" phenomena of the celiac artery by the median arcuate ligament

celiac artery distribution. This subsequently deprives the midgut of necessary blood flow and causes the classic postprandial abdominal symptoms of MALS [9]. There is no consensus as to the true mechanism of ischemia in MALS pathology, and multiple theories provide helpful anatomic explanations for various elements of MALS pathology.

Neurogenic Theory: Compression of the Celiac Ganglion

A neuropathic component has also been postulated to contribute to MALS through compression of the celiac ganglion and plexus [5, 10]. There is a wide range of variations in plexus morphology, interconnections, and location [4]. The celiac plexus rests superiorly on the CA, and there is a possibility for impingement of the ganglia by the MAL, which could result in a myriad of abdominal symptoms from sympathetic overstimulation of pain fibers. This theory has been evaluated through diagnostic testing with celiac plexus nerve blocks and interventions targeting the celiac ganglion, rather than revascularization. Several of these patients experience symptomatic relief, albeit transiently [11, 12]. In addition, there are reports of patients who have undergone laparoscopic median arcuate ligament release (MALR) with persistent stenosis of greater than 70% postoperatively who have symptom relief [13]. These studies suggest there likely is a neurogenic component to the etiology of MALS in select patients. As such, many surgeons, including these authors, advocate for routine celiac ganglion splanchnicectomy during MALR procedures.

Conclusion

In summary, MALS is a rare but often debilitating condition that results in chronic, unrelenting postprandial epigastric pain. Its cause is incompletely understood but may be due to a combination of vasculogenic and neurogenic causes related to compression of the celiac trunk and ganglia by the MAL. Knowledge of this pathophysiology is critical to understanding the diagnostic workup and subsequent therapeutic options for this challenging group of patients.

References

1. Moore, et al. Moore clinically oriented anatomy. 8th ed. Philadelphia: Wolters Kluwer Health; 2018.
2. Loukas M, Pinyard J, Vaid S, Kinsella C, Tariq A, Tubbs RS. Clinical anatomy of celiac artery compression syndrome: a review. Clin Anat. 2007;20:612–7.
3. Lindner HH, Kemprud E. A clinicoanatomical study of the arcuate ligament of the diaphragm. Arch Surg. 1971;103:600–5. https://doi.org/10.1001/archsurg.1971.01350110102016.

4. Bech FR. Celiac artery compression syndromes. Surg Clin N Am. 1997;77:409–24. https://doi.org/10.1016/S0039-6109(05)70558-2.
5. Katz-Summercorn A, Bridger J. A cadaveric study of the anatomical variation of the origins of the celiac trunk and the superior mesenteric artery: a role in median arcuate ligament syndrome? Clin Anat. 2013;26:971–4. https://doi.org/10.1002/CA.22243.
6. Dyches RP, Eaton KJ, Smith HF. The roles of celiac trunk angle and vertebral origin in median arcuate ligament syndrome. Diagnostics. 2020;10:20076. https://doi.org/10.3390/diagnostics10020076.
7. Reuter SR, Bernstein EF. The anatomic basis for respiratory variation in median arcuate ligament compression of the celiac artery. Surgery. 1973;73:381–5.
8. Kornblith PL, Boley SJ, Whitehouse BS. Anatomy of the splanchnic circulation. Surg Clin N Am. 1992;72:1–30.
9. Watson WC, Sadikali F. Celiac axis compression. Experience with 20 patients and a critical appraisal of the syndrome. Ann Intern Med. 1977;86:278–84. https://doi.org/10.7326/0003-4819-86-3-278.
10. Tribble CG, Harman PK, Mentzer RM. Celiac artery compression syndrome: report of a case and review of current opinion. Vasc Endovasc Surg. 1986;20:120–9.
11. Sultan S, Hynes N. PS160. Management of median arcuate ligament syndrome (MALS) with decompression and Coeliac Ganglion Sympathectomy (CGS) for chronic mesenteric ischaemia (CMI). Procedural, clinical and enduring results with quality-adjusted time spent without symptoms of disease and toxicity of treatment (Q-TWiST). J Vasc Surg. 2010;51:62S. https://doi.org/10.1016/j.jvs.2010.02.288.
12. Selvaraj BJ, Joshi M, Weber G, Yarmush J. Celiac plexus block as a diagnostic tool in suspected pediatric median arcuate ligament syndrome. Local Reg Anesth. 2019;12:15–8. https://doi.org/10.2147/LRA.S191851.
13. Weber JM, Boules M, Fong K, Abraham B, Bena J, El-Hayek K, Kroh M, Michael Park W. Median arcuate ligament syndrome is not a vascular disease. Ann Vasc Surg. 2016;30:13. https://doi.org/10.1016/j.avsg.2015.07.013.

Chapter 3
Anatomy of Median Arcuate Ligament Syndrome

Amanda Belluzzi, Aida K. Sarcon, Omar M. Ghanem, and Todd E. Rasmussen

Introduction

The median arcuate ligament arises from the union of the right and left crus of the diaphragm overlying the aortic hiatus. The celiac trunk (CT) is the first major branch of the abdominal aorta (AA) and typically trifurcates into the left gastric, common hepatic, and splenic arteries. The inferior phrenic arteries lie in close vicinity to the CT, often arising from the CT or sometimes off the AA. The celiac ganglion, which many believe to be at least partially responsible for the symptoms caused by MALS, is often located on either side or directly anterior to the celiac artery.

A. Belluzzi
Department of General Surgery, Rovigo Hospital, Rovigo, Italy

Department of Metabolic and Abdominal Wall Reconstructive Surgery, Mayo Clinic, Rochester, MN, USA

A. K. Sarcon
Department of Surgery, Mayo Clinic, Rochester, MN, USA

O. M. Ghanem
Department of Surgery, Mayo Clinic, Rochester, MN, USA

T. E. Rasmussen (✉)
Department of Vascular Surgery, Mayo Clinic, Rochester, MN, USA
e-mail: rasmussen.todd@mayo.edu

D. Shouhed et al. (eds.), *Median Arcuate Ligament Syndrome*,
https://doi.org/10.1007/978-3-031-80740-4_3

Celiac Trunk

The CT originates from the ventral aspect of the aorta at the level of T12–L1 vertebrae. Its historical description mentions a main trunk that branches into the common hepatic artery (CHA), left gastric artery (LGA), and splenic artery (SA); this trifurcation pattern was first described by Haller in 1756 as "Tripus Haller" [1]. A true classical trifurcation occurs when all three branches of the CT divide at the same site. A false trifurcation occurs when the LGA branches off as an individual collateral, leaving the CT to divide terminally into the SA and CHA (Fig. 3.1). The absence of the celiac trunk with the origin of the three arteries separately from the aorta is a rare entity that is reported in 0.38% to 2.6% of cases in the literature [3].

Anatomic variations of the CT can be explained by the Mackay Arch and Tandler theories. According to the first, the distribution of the embryonic aortic branches is metameric. Every metamere gives rise to three pairs of branches which unite in a posterior, lateral, and anterior or visceral arch. The visceral arches then evolve into a single metameric median digestive artery. The 10th, 11th, and 12th metameric arteries form the LGA, SA, and CHA, respectively, while the 13th metameric artery gives rise to the superior mesenteric artery (SMA) [4].

According to the Tandler theory, the embryological origin of the splanchnic vessels stems from developmental changes occurring in ventral segmental arteries 10–22. As the embryo begins its maturation process, the roots of the 11th and 12th ventral segmental arteries regress and gradually disappear. However, the 10th

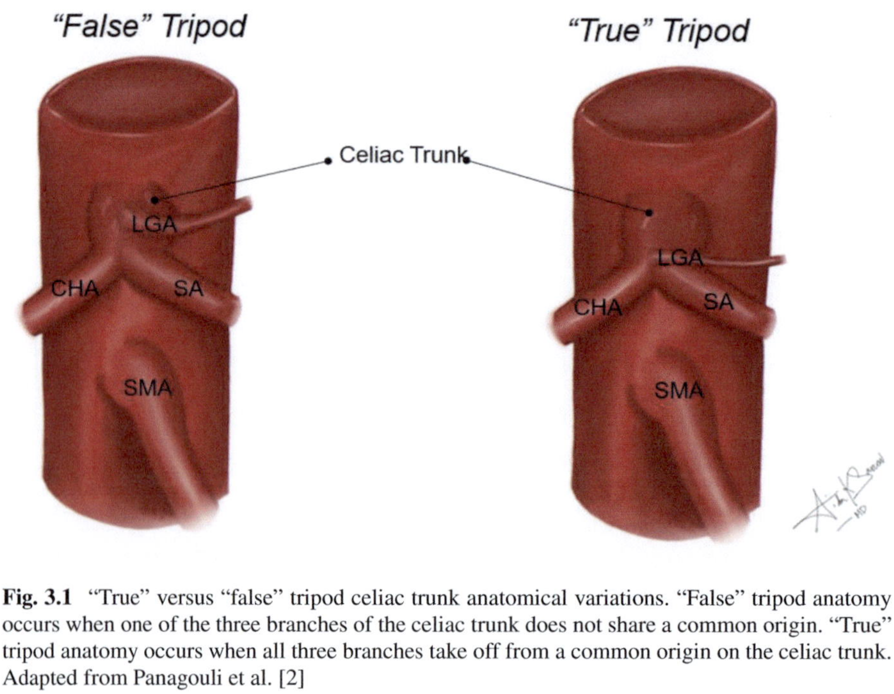

Fig. 3.1 "True" versus "false" tripod celiac trunk anatomical variations. "False" tripod anatomy occurs when one of the three branches of the celiac trunk does not share a common origin. "True" tripod anatomy occurs when all three branches take off from a common origin on the celiac trunk. Adapted from Panagouli et al. [2]

ventral segmental artery persists as the CT, and the SMA develops from the persistent 13th segmental artery. During this process, a ventral longitudinal anastomosis may remain intact, serving as a direct anastomosis between the celiac artery and the SMA [5].

Many authors have defined several classifications for variations of the CT. However, even when widely accepted classifications are taken as a theoretical basis to refer to, many new variants are reported [6]. The first classification of anatomical variations of the celiac trunk was proposed by Adachi and Hasebe in 1928, which consists of six different types: hepatogastrosplenic trunk (HGST, 86%), the true tripus Halleri configuration, hepatosplenic trunk (HST, 8%), (3) hepatosplenomesenteric trunk (HSMT, 1%), celiacomesenteric trunk (CMT, 1.5%); hepatomesenteric trunk (HMT, 0.5%), and gastrosplenic trunk (GST, 3%). These variations were found after Adachi performed and documented on 252 dissected cadavers [7].

In the literature, the classic trifurcation pattern of the CT was reported between 74 and 93% [6, 8], while the frequency of the HST has been reported between 2.3 and 8.3% [9]. Alternatively, the bifurcation of the CT occurs in approximately 11% of the general population, where one branch of the trunk is absent or develops independently from the abdominal aorta (AA) (Figs. 3.2 and 3.3). Depending on the two arteries emerging from the CT, this variation can take on different nomenclatures, such as, the hepatosplenic, hepatogastric, and gastrosplenic [10]. Other variations mentioned in the literature include quadrifurcation, pentafurcation, hexafurcation,

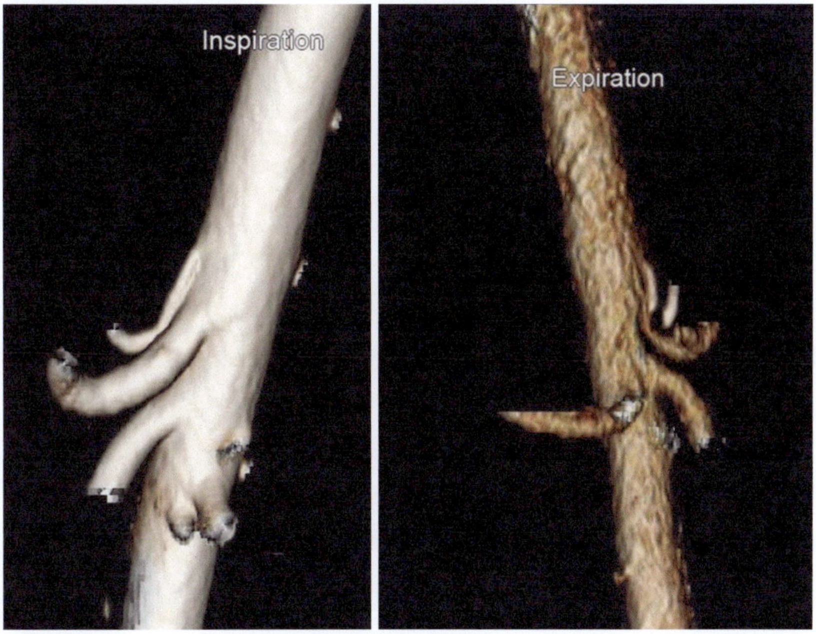

Figs. 3.2 and 3.3 Left gastric artery arising from the aorta on CT scan inspiration and expiration phase

and agenesis of the CT (Fig. 3.4) [11–13]. The absence of the celiac trunk is a rare variation in which all three major branches arise independently from the AA. Most radiologic and cadaveric collections have recorded instances of this variation, ranging from 0.1% to 2.6% [14]. Morita's classification was the first to include the absence of a celiac trunk in its types, which included type 1, normal celiac trunk; type 2, hepatosplenic trunk; type 3, gastro-splenic trunk; type 4, hepatogastric trunk; and type 5, absent celiac trunk (Fig. 3.5) [15].

Regarding CMT, its prevalence varies between 0.3% and 0.62%. Incomplete CMT is seen between 0.16% and 0.37% [16], while a celiacomesenteric anastomosis is found between 0.04% and 0.13% (Fig. 3.6) [17]. Among the acknowledged anatomic possibilities of celiacomesenteric anastomoses, it is worth mentioning the arc of Bühler (AOB), a direct celiacomesenteric anastomosis, which was described by Bühler in 1904 [18, 19]. The AOB is described as the remnant segment of Tandler's longitudinal anterior anastomosis between the embryonic splanchnic branches of the abdominal aorta, which account for the celiacomesenteric and intermesenteric anastomoses in adults (Fig. 3.7) [4, 13, 20], with a prevalence ranging

Fig. 3.4 Quadrifurcation of the CT

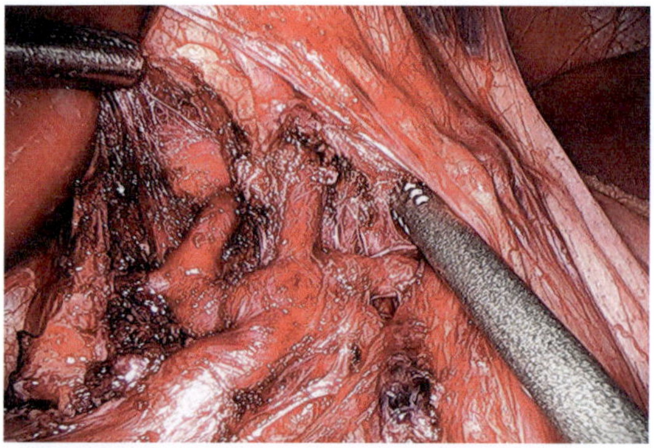

Fig. 3.5 Hepatogastric variation with the absence of the splenic artery from the CT

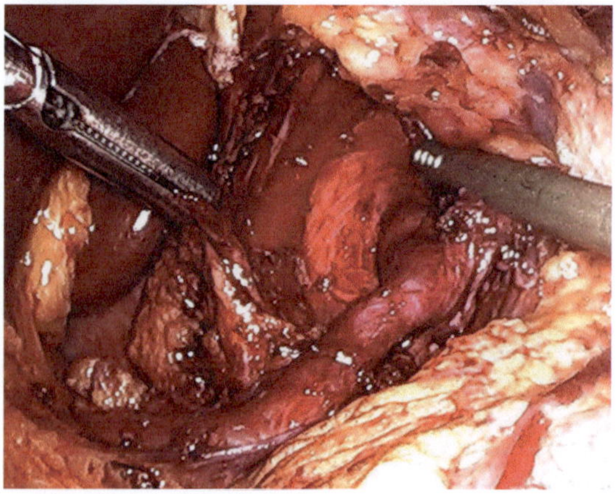

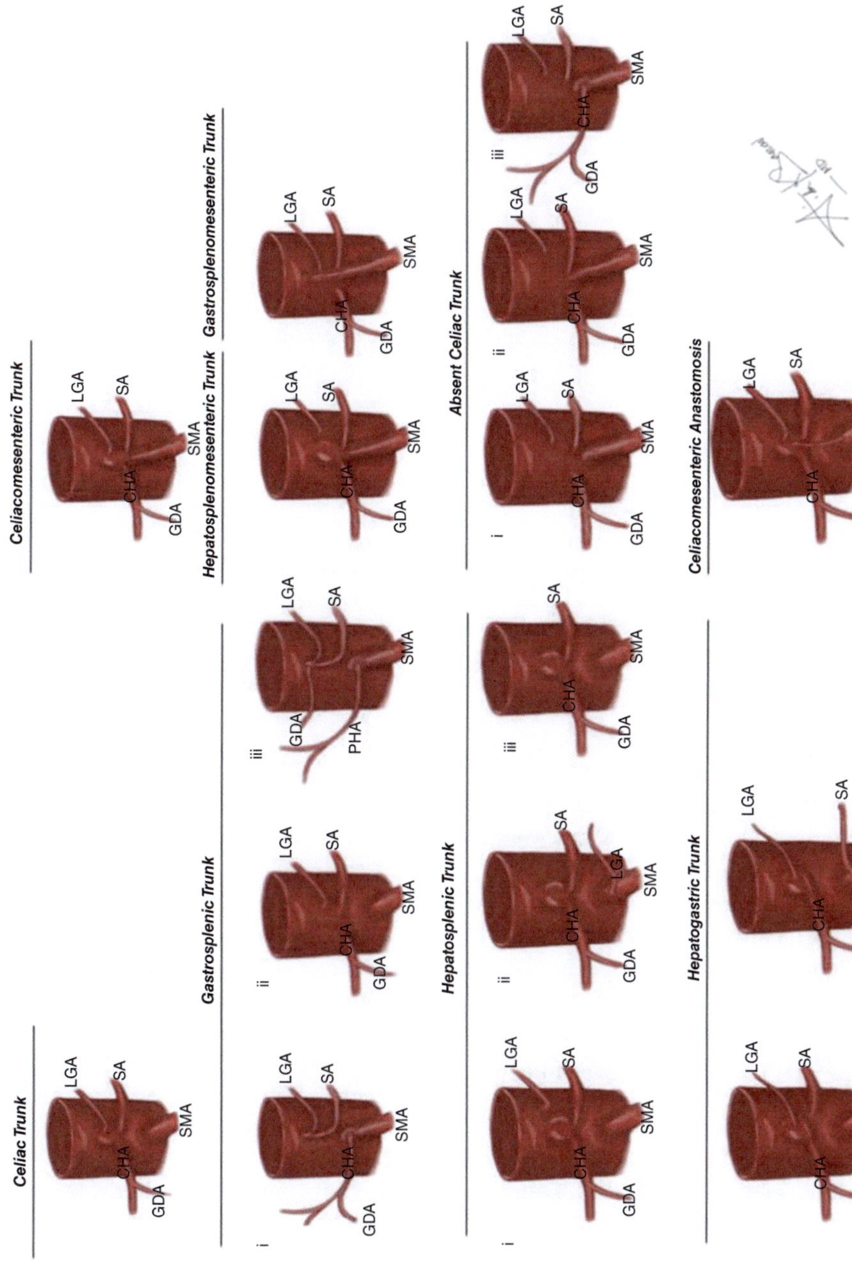

Fig. 3.6 Various types of celiac trunk variations from 17,391 cases with celiac trunk mutations adapted from Whitley et al. [17]

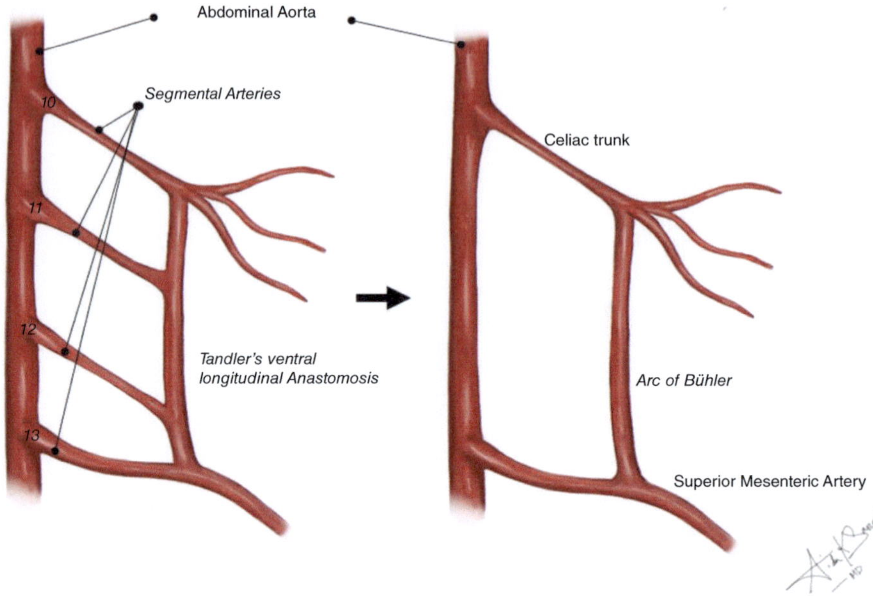

Fig. 3.7 Tandler's theory (formation of the Arc of Bühler). The 10th to 13th segmental arteries join Tandler's ventral longitudinal anastomosis. Normally, there is a regression of the 11th to 12th segmental arteries and a segment (between the 10th and the 13th arteries) of the longitudinal anastomosis. The persistence of Tandler's anastomosis will form the Arc of Bühler, which then unites the celiac trunk (or its branches) with the superior mesenteric artery adapted from Manta et al. [13]

between 1% and 4% and an average of 1.7% based on a recent systematic review [21]. The importance of the AOB is related to its role in supplying the branches of the CT from the SMA in case of CT stenosis. Moreover, the AOB, if present as a definitive vasculature, can provide collateral circulation to some organs supplied by the pancreaticoduodenal artery (PDA) [22]. Other common classifications employed for the description of the CT and its variants are those described by Michels [23], Hiatt [24], Panagouli [2], and Prakash [25].

According to the most recent classification by Marco-Clement et al., branching of the CT can be divided into four main types: complete (type I), incomplete (type II), no celiac trunk (type III), and celiacomesenteric trunk (type IV) [26]. The least frequent type of celiac trunk branching pattern is type III, in which all branches originate directly from the aorta or from its branches. This type of variation was reported by Vandamme et al. in 1.3% of 156 anatomical specimens [27]. In the recent work of Bilek et al., the "New Celiac Trunk Classification" developed by Dilli Babu et al. was used [28]. Dilli Babu et al. initially defined six main types and 16 subtypes [29]. Later, the same authors published a new paper reporting 18 subtypes [30].

Inferior Phrenic Arteries

The right and left inferior phrenic arteries (IPAs) typically originate as early branches from the abdominal aorta. In addition to the esophagus, stomach, spleen, liver, diaphragm, and adjacent structures, the inferior phrenic arteries supply the adrenal glands via a branch known as the superior suprarenal artery. The posterior branches of both IPAs run lateral to the diaphragmatic crus and can anastomose with the musculophrenic artery and the lower posterior intercostal arteries [31, 32]. Several authors have reported that IPAs may arise from various sites, such as the abdominal aorta (46.8% cases), celiac trunk (46.1% cases), and renal arteries (1.47% cases). In rare cases, the IPAs may arise from the splenic, superior mesenteric, or gonadal arteries [33–35].

In a recent systematic review and meta-analysis by Whitley et al., a common inferior phrenic artery (CIPA) was reported to have a pooled prevalence of 24.2%, while left and right IPAs had a separate origin in 75.8% of cases. When originating separately, the aorta and the celiac trunk were the most common sites of origin with a reported pooled prevalence of 57.2% and 41.3%, respectively. Other rare sites of origin included the left gastric artery, the right and left renal artery, and the left middle adrenal artery with an overall combined prevalence of 1% [33].

The right inferior phrenic artery (RIPA) was reported to originate from the aorta, the celiac trunk, the right renal artery, and the left gastric artery with a prevalence of 49.6%, 35.7%, 10.3%, and 2.07%, respectively. Other rarer sites of origin were reported, which include the common hepatic artery, right hepatic artery, proper hepatic artery, SMA, dorsal pancreatic artery, and a common trunk made of adrenal and gonadal arteries [33]. On the other hand, the left inferior phrenic artery (LIPA) was reported to originate from the aorta, the celiac trunk, the left renal artery, and the left gastric artery with a prevalence of 46.8%, 46.1%, 1.47%, and 1.07%, respectively. Other less frequent origins included the hepatic arteries, left middle-adrenal artery, and right inferior phrenic artery [33].

Both right and left inferior phrenic arteries can present as accessory vessels originating from the abdominal aorta, left gastric artery, celiac trunk, or right inferior phrenic artery itself [31, 36–38]. Precise detailed knowledge of the anatomy of the inferior phrenic arteries is paramount when performing MALS surgery, since iatrogenic bleeding has frequently been reported as a possible intraoperative complication [39].

Median Arcuate Ligament

The median arcuate ligament is a musculofibrous arciform structure uniting both sides of the diaphragmatic crura anterior to the aortic hiatus at the level of T12. The diaphragmatic crura are attached to the anterior surfaces of vertebrae L1 to L4 on the right and left from vertebrae L2 to L3. The crura unite with the median arcuate ligament after crossing upward and anteriorly to the aortic hiatus. It has been postulated by several authors that in 10–24% of the population, the MAL crosses the aorta at an atypically inferior anatomic position with subsequent compression of the CT and ganglion [40, 41]. This low-lying position of the MAL can be explained by the differential growth of the anterior and posterior regions of the embryo when the septum transversum starts to descend, whereby week eight it reaches the level of the thoracic vertebrae. At this point, the two crura (legs) of the diaphragm develop as muscular extensions attaching to the lateral side of the lumbar vertebrae [42, 43].

A study by Lindner et al. showed that the origin of the (CT) origin was at or above the level of the MAL in 33% of patients [44]. However, it was unclear whether compression of the CT was related to a higher level of origin of the CT, an inferior extension of the diaphragm, or a combination of the two. Other authors considered the angle of origin of the CT off the aorta to be the best indicator to evaluate the compression of the CT. It was also suggested that acute deviation of the left and right diaphragmatic crura may lead to compression of the CT by the MAL. Eventually, they concluded MALS patients are more prone to having an inferiorly positioned or elongated diaphragm than a high CT in relation to a more acute CT angle of origin and subsequent increased occurrence of MAL/CT overlap [43].

Celiac Ganglion

The celiac plexus consists of paired ganglia interconnected by nerve fibers, which are located on either side of the celiac artery [45]. Although its position varies, several authors have reported that 94% of the celiac ganglia are located at the level of T12 or L1 [46–49]. The left celiac ganglion is approximately 0.9 cm caudal to the CT, while the right celiac ganglion is only 0.6 cm caudal to the CT [48]. The mean size of the celiac ganglion is about 2.7 cm, ranging from 0.5 to 4.5 cm [46, 48, 50–53].

Both ganglia can be identified during diagnostic abdominal computed tomography; however, the left celiac ganglion is typically better visualized than the right. This could be explained by the limited space between the IVC and the right diaphragmatic crus. In relation to shape, the right and left ganglia demonstrate a characteristic discoid or multilobulated configuration that resembles the limbs of the adjacent adrenal gland. A more comprehensive report highlights that they are irregular in appearance, varying between round, oval, triangular, and crescent shape [45, 46, 54, 55]. On axial CT images, the left celiac ganglion is consistently seen anteromedial to the left adrenal gland, between the adrenal gland and the diaphragmatic crus, while the right celiac ganglion is often located between the inferior vena cava (IVC) and the right diaphragmatic crus, anteromedial to the right adrenal gland and posteromedial to the IVC [56]. The correct identification of the celiac ganglia is paramount not only during the meticulous layer-by-layer surgical dissection of the ganglionic fibers but also during celiac plexus block (CPB) to avoid organ penetration and bleeding [53, 57].

Conclusion

The art of surgery is dictated by the mastery of anatomy. The enclosed, deep region, where the celiac trunk resides within the abdomen, accentuates the importance of anatomy when performing surgery for MALS. Familiarization with both normal and variant anatomy of the celiac trunk and ganglia will make for a safer, more efficient, and more effective operation with a potential reduction of intraoperative and postoperative complications.

References

1. Haller VA. Icones anatomicae in quibus aliquae partes corporis humani declineate proponuntur et arteriarum potissimum historia continetur. Gottingen: Vandenhoeck; 1765.
2. Panagouli E, Venieratos D, Lolis E, Skandalakis P. Variations in the anatomy of the celiac trunk: a systematic review and clinical implications. Ann Anat. 2013;195(6):501–11.
3. Covantsev S, Uzdenov R, Mazuruc N, Turovets D, Belic O. Absent celiac trunk and unusual arterial anatomy of the upper abdomen: into the deep. Folia Med. 2023;65(3):500–7.
4. Michalinos A, Schizas D, Ntourakis D, et al. Arc of Bühler: the surgical significance of a rare anatomical variation. Surg Radiol Anat. 2019;41(5):575–81.
5. Tandler J. Über die Varietäten der Arteria coeliaca und deren Entwickelung. Anat Hefte. 1904;25(2):473–500.
6. Türkyılmaz Z, Kula O, Çelik AO, Demirel T, Günay B. Evaluation of celiac artery and common hepatic artery variations by CT-angiography and new classification model. Surg Radiol Anat. 2023;45(8):1037–47.
7. Adachi B, Hasebe K. Das Arteriensystem der Japaner. Kaiserlich-japanische Universität zu Kyoto, in kommission bei "Maruzen Co". Kyoto and Tokyo; 1928.
8. Sureka B, Mittal MK, Mittal A, Sinha M, Bhambri NK, Thukral BB. Variations of celiac axis, common hepatic artery and its branches in 600 patients. Indian J Radiol Imaging. 2013;23(3):223–33.
9. Song SB, Mittal MK, Mittal A, Sinha M, Bhambri NK, Thukral BB. Variations of celiac axis, common hepatic artery and its branches in 600 patients. Indian J Radiol Imaging. 2013;23(3):223–33.
10. Santos PV, Barbosa ABM, Targino VA, et al. Anatomical variations of the celiac trunk: a systematic review. Arq Bras Cir Dig. 2018;31:e1403.
11. Rusu MC, Jianu AM, Dinca D, Manta BA. Quadrifurcation variants of the celiac trunk. Ann Vasc Surg. 2021;73:303–13.
12. Rusu MC, Jianu AM, Manta BA, Hostiuc S. Aortic origins of the celiac trunk and superior mesenteric artery. Diagnostics. 2021;11(6):1111.
13. Manta BA, Rusu MC, Jianu AM, Ilie AC. Hexafurcated coeliac trunks, trifurcated common hepatic artery, and a new variant of the arc of Bühler. Folia Morphol (Warsz). 2022;81(2):365–71.
14. Fahmy D, Sadek H. A case of absent celiac trunk: case report and review of the literature. Egypt J Radiol Nucl Med. 2015;46(4):1021–4.
15. Morita M. Reports and conception of three anomalous cases on the area of the celiac and the superior mesenteric arteries. Igaku Kenkyu. 1935;9:1993–2006.
16. Cankal F, Kaya M, Guner MA. Evaluation of celiac trunk, hepatic artery variations, and their collateral arteries by multi-slice computed tomography. Sisli Etfal Hastan Tip Bul. 2021;55(2):217–23.

17. Whitley A, Oliverius M, Kocián P, Havlůj L, Gürlich R, Kachlík D. Variations of the celiac trunk investigated by multidetector computed tomography: Systematic review and meta-analysis with clinical correlations. Clin Anat. 2020;33:1249–62.
18. Bühler A. Über eine Anastomose zwischen den Stämmen der Art. coeliaca und der Art. mesenterica superior. Gegenbaurs Morphol Jahrb. 1904;32:185–8.
19. Saad WE, Davies MG, Sahler L, Lee D, Patel N, Kitanosono T, et al. Arc of Buhler: incidence and diameter in asymptomatic individuals. Vasc Endovasc Surg. 2005;39:347–9.
20. Rusu MC, Vlad M, Voinea LM, Curca GC, Sisu AM. Detailed anatomy of a left accessory aberrant colic artery. Surg Radiol Anat. 2008;30:595–9.
21. Kowalczyk KA, Pękala J, Kawzowicz M, Pękala PA, Tomaszewski KA. The meta-analysis and systematic review of prevalence and clinical anatomy of the arc of Buhler. Sci Rep. 2023;13:9183.
22. Abouzaid KA, Lichtenberg AB, Karim AY, Stack ER, Algoul M, Imam A, Macpherson AA, Chanthanivong CV. A unique arc of Bühler variant connecting the arteries of the foregut, midgut, and hindgut and its surgical significance. Cureus. 2023;15(7):e42611.
23. Michels NA. Newer anatomy of the liver and its variant blood supply and collateral circulation. Am J Surg. 1966;112:337–47.
24. Hiatt JR, Gabbay J, Busuttil RW. Surgical anatomy of the hepatic arteries in 1000 cases. Ann Surg. 1994;220(1):50–2.
25. Prakash RT, Mokhasi V, Geethanjali BS, Sivacharan PV, Shashirekha M. Coeliac trunk and its branches: anatomical variations and clinical implications. Singapore Med J. 2012;53:329–31.
26. Marco-Clement I, Martinez-Barco A, Ahumada N, et al. Anatomical variations of the celiac trunk: cadaveric and radiological study. Surg Radiol Anat. 2016;38(4):501–10.
27. Vandamme JP, Bonte J. The branches of the celiac trunk. Acta Anat. 1985;122(2):110–4.
28. Bilek E, Keven A, Arslan AG. Comprehensive analysis of splenic artery variations using computed tomography angiography: development of the IPALGEA classification system. Surg Radiol Anat. 2024;46(3):363–76.
29. Dilli Babu E, Khrab P. Coeliac trunk variations: review with proposed new classification. Int J Anat Res. 2013;3:165–70.
30. Dilli Babu E, Kalyanasundaram S, Indiran V, et al. Newly proposed classification of celiac artery variations based on embryology and correlation with computed tomography angiography. Pol J Radiol. 2022;87(1):563–73.
31. Piao DX, Ohtsuka A, Murakami T. Typology of abdominal arteries, with special reference to inferior phrenic arteries and their esophageal branches. Acta Med Austriaca. 1998;52(4):189–96.
32. Pulakunta T, Potu B, Gorantla V, et al. The origin of the inferior phrenic artery: a study in 32 South Indian cadavers with a review of the literature. J Vasc Bras. 2007;6(3):225–30.
33. Whitley A, Křeček J, Kachlík D. The inferior phrenic arteries: a systematic review and meta-analysis. Ann Anat. 2021;235:151679.
34. Gwon DI, Ko G-Y, Yoon H-K, et al. Inferior phrenic artery: anatomy, variations, pathologic conditions, and interventional management. RadioGraphics. 2007;27(3):687–705.
35. Kahn PC. Selective angiography of the inferior phrenic arteries. Radiology. 1967;88(1):1–8.
36. Ozbülbül NI, Yurdakul M, Tola M. Does the right inferior phrenic artery have a supplying role in liver cirrhosis without hepatocellular carcinoma? A64-slice CT study. Diagn Interv Radiol. 2011;17:239–42.
37. Cauldwell EW, Anson BJ. The visceral branches of the abdominal aorta: topographical relationships. Am J Anat. 1943;73:27–57.
38. Pick JW, Anson BJ. The inferior phrenic artery: origin and suprarenal branches. Anat Rec. 1940;78:413–27.
39. Belluzzi A, Salame M, Abi Mosleh K, Rasmussen TE, Kendrick ML, Ghanem OM. Laparoscopic median arcuate ligament release: surgical technique and clinical outcomes. Surg Laparosc Endosc Percutan Tech. 2024;34(1):74–9.

40. Sultan S, Hynes N, Elsafty N, Tawfick W. Eight years experience in the management of median arcuate ligament syndrome by decompression, celiac ganglion sympathectomy, and selective revascularization. Vasc Endovasc Surg. 2013;47(8):614–9.
41. Storm J, Kerr E, Kennedy P. Rare complications of a low lying median arcuate coeliac ligament. Ulster Med J. 2015;84(2):107–9.
42. Moore KL, Dalley AF, Moore A. Clinically oriented anatomy. 8th ed. Philadelphia: Lippincott Williams & Wilkins; 2017. p. 1–1168.
43. Dyches RP, Eaton KJ, Smith HF. The roles of celiac trunk angle and vertebral origin in median arcuate ligament syndrome. Diagnostics. 2020;10(2):76.
44. Lindner HH, Kemprud E. A clinicoanatomical study of the arcuate ligament of the diaphragm. Arch Surg. 1971;103:600–5.
45. du Plessis M, Loukas M. A comprehensive study of the abdominal ganglia part 1: celiac, phrenic and superior mesenteric ganglia. Clin Anat. 2022;35(7):998–1006.
46. Zhang XM, Zhao QH, Zeng NL, et al. The celiac ganglia: anatomic study using MRI in cadavers. AJR Am J Roentgenol. 2006;186(6):1520–3.
47. Loukas M, Klaassen Z, Merbs W, Tubbs RS, Gielecki J, Zurada A. A review of the thoracic splanchnic nerves and celiac ganglia. Clin Anat. 2010;23(5):512–22.
48. Titton RL, Lucey BC, Gervais DA, Boland GW, Mueller PR. Celiac plexus block: a palliative tool underused by radiologists. AJR Am J Roentgenol. 2002;179(3):633–6.
49. Kambadakone A, Thabet A, Gervais DA, Mueller PR, Arellano RS. CT-guided celiac plexus neurolysis: a review of anatomy, indications, technique, and tips for successful treatment. Radiographics. 2011;31(6):1599–621.
50. De Cicco M, Matovic M, Balestreri L, Fracasso A, Morassut S, Testa V. Single-needle celiac plexus block: is needle tip position critical in patients with no regional anatomic distortions? Anesthesiology. 1997;87(6):1301–8.
51. Loukas PID. Coeliac plexus neurolysis. Best Pract Res Clin Gastroenterol. 2009;23(5):761–6.
52. De Cicco M, Matovic M, Bortolussi R, et al. Celiac plexus block: injectate spread and pain relief in patients with regional anatomic distortions. Anesthesiology. 2001;94(4):561–5.
53. Penman ID, Gilbert D. Basic technique for celiac plexus block/neurolysis. Gastrointest Endosc. 2009;69(2 suppl):S163–5.
54. Ward EM, Rorie DK, Nauss LA, Bahn RC. The celiac ganglia in man: normal anatomic variations. Anesth Analg. 1979;58:461–5.
55. Paz Z, Rosen A. The human celiac ganglion and its splanchnic nerves. Acta Anat. 1989;136(2):129–33.
56. Wang ZJ, Webb EM, Westphalen AC, Coakley FV, Yeh BM. Multi-detector row computed tomographic appearance of celiac ganglia. J Comput Assist Tomogr. 2010;34(3):343–7.
57. Yang IY, Oraee S, Viejo C, et al. Computed tomography celiac trunk topography relating to celiac plexus block. Reg Anesth Pain Med. 2011;36:21–5.

Chapter 4
Symptoms, Presentation, and Differential Diagnosis of Median Arcuate Ligament Syndrome

Leif Sorensen, Jennifer Curti, and Nathan G. Richards

Introduction

Median arcuate ligament syndrome (MALS) presents a formidable diagnostic challenge in clinical practice, often eluding recognition and leading to misdiagnosis. Characterized by a compression of the celiac artery and the interposing celiac plexus fibers and ganglia, MALS manifests through a spectrum of symptoms, often debilitating in nature. In fact, an infrequent or mild complaint of symptoms may favor a different diagnosis or perhaps a presentation that does not obviate surgery, especially if there isn't a compromise in the patient's quality of life.

Most patients complain of postprandial epigastric pain often radiating to the left upper quadrant along the left subcostal margin and nausea, leading to sitophobia and resulting in significant weight loss. Other common symptoms include exercise intolerance, early satiety, bloating and difficulty breathing. Despite its rarity, MALS is frequently overlooked, underappreciated, or misunderstood, contributing to delays in diagnosis and suboptimal symptom management. MALS symptoms can be nonspecific and frequently overlap with other gastrointestinal and psychiatric disorders, leading to confusion, redundant testing, and frustration with consistently "normal" results. This lack of obvious markers and indisputable evidence

L. Sorensen
Department of Surgery, University of Utah, Salt Lake City, UT, USA

J. Curti
Division of General Surgery, Intermountain Medical Group, Intermountain Health, LDS Hospital, Salt Lake City, UT, USA

N. G. Richards (✉)
Department of Surgery, University of Utah, Salt Lake City, UT, USA

Division of General Surgery, Intermountain Medical Group, Intermountain Health, LDS Hospital, Salt Lake City, UT, USA
e-mail: Nathan.richards@imail.org

D. Shouhed et al. (eds.), *Median Arcuate Ligament Syndrome*,
https://doi.org/10.1007/978-3-031-80740-4_4

underscores the importance of heightened clinical suspicion and a comprehensive diagnostic approach. These tools enable clinicians to navigate diagnostic challenges more effectively, ultimately improving the accuracy of diagnosis, appropriateness of intervention, patient outcomes, and quality of life for patients, their families, and care teams.

Symptoms of Median Arcuate Ligament Syndrome (MALS)

While ischemia is often presumed to be the primary driver of symptoms, emerging evidence, particularly over the last decade, suggests that neurogenic compression of the celiac plexus may play the primary role in symptomatology [1–3]. In this scenario, the ligament is like a blacksmith's hammer, and the artery is like the anvil. The celiac plexus nerves are the metal being molded, changed, and compressed. Unfortunately, this maladaptive compression renders the nerves thickened, damaged, fibrotic, and unreliable. As these nerves are responsible for initiating and driving digestion, their damage renders the process ineffective, often resulting in unintelligible signals moving from the ganglia of the celiac plexus to the brainstem. The brainstem's default mechanism to stop the broken signals from being generated is to cause the patient to feel epigastric pain and nausea. Pain and nausea result in eating cessation, and the celiac plexus signals dissipate. Notably, MALS patients often present with progressive symptoms. Pain and nausea usually begin with certain foods or consistencies. With time, most patients note that almost all foods and liquids can elicit symptoms. They realize that it is not what they are eating, but rather, how much. Ultimately, these patients note that symptoms evolve to a standard baseline pain that builds throughout the day and is exacerbated with any oral intake.

The hallmark feature of median arcuate ligament syndrome (MALS) is epigastric abdominal pain [4, 5], particularly postprandial pain, characterized by a dull or aching discomfort in the epigastric region following meals. The true prevalence of MALS is challenging to ascertain because of its variable clinical presentation [6]. However, in a case series involving 43 individuals who underwent surgical treatment for MALS, 91% presented with abdominal pain, 40% experienced weight loss, and 30% reported nausea as clinical symptoms [7]. Many patients note that the pain is improved or potentially alleviated by drawing the knees to the chest or leaning forward [8, 9]. Patients often describe the pain as stabbing, squeezing, or pressure-like in nature, with variations in intensity and duration. The onset of pain shortly after eating is a characteristic feature, with symptoms often presenting within 15 min of oral intake and persisting for hours after, significantly impacting daily activities and dietary habits. With advanced disease, it is common for the pain to become constant with postprandial exacerbation.

As outlined previously, dysautonomia and inhibitory oversight from the brainstem also often result in chronic nausea [10–12]. Interestingly, vomiting tends to be less prominent, although certainly not absent. The nausea of MALS is gnawing, omnipresent, and worse with eating. Most patients describe it as always and immediately feeling full. The ineffective celiac plexus coordination of the stomach and potentially other digestive organs can impair nutrient absorption and gastrointestinal function, leading to persistent nausea [13–15].

Epigastric pain and unrelenting nausea often combine to promote unintended weight loss in patients with MALS because of sitophobia. Patients typically report a decreased appetite and aversion to food due to associated symptoms. Most patients will either recount eating very small meals to minimize symptoms or eating one big meal to only suffer through the pain once a day. These patients are almost always at risk of protein deficiency. In addition, there is a significant correlation between food fear and more formal eating disorders, including anorexia nervosa. It is critical to understand the etiology of their symptoms well to tease out contributing factors. Addressing nutritional deficiencies and effectively managing symptoms are crucial components of MALS management to improve overall patient outcomes.

Individuals afflicted with MALS often report intolerance to food and liquid intake. Symptoms such as early satiety, bloating, and postprandial discomfort indicate compromised digestive function, contributing to diminished appetite and potential nutritional deficiencies. Patients may experience discomfort or pain shortly after eating, leading to the avoidance of certain foods or smaller meal portions. Understanding the impact of food intolerance on dietary habits and nutritional status is crucial for clinicians to tailor management strategies accordingly.

Frequently, patients with MALS present with pain and nausea related to exercise and activity. It is common for patients to describe exacerbation of epigastric pain and potentiation of nausea with strenuous activity, certain repetitive movements, and exercise. Some young patients diagnosed with MALS have a history of being involved in club, high school, or college athletics. In these patients, a familiar story is that symptoms worsened with activity duration, and the patient was forced to reduce activity; stop playing, either temporarily or permanently; and lose scholarship funds or opportunities.

The symptoms [6] of MALS encompass a spectrum of manifestations that significantly impair the quality of life of affected individuals. Recognizing these symptoms is paramount for accurate diagnosis and effective management. Clinicians who understand the diverse symptoms can provide comprehensive care to individuals with MALS, optimizing outcomes and improving overall well-being.

Presentation

The presentation of MALS is characterized by a constellation of symptoms and diagnostic challenges, contributing to delays in diagnosis and management. Most patients have been suffering for years before reaching a diagnosis and often present with severe weight loss. It is not uncommon for patients to be on medical leave from work or school, retracting themselves from most social activity, and suffering from a feeling of depression and despair leading to suicidal ideations [16–18].

One of the defining features of MALS is the prolonged duration of symptoms that are often ambiguous or easily attributed to other causes. Many patients or their families will recount a history of gastrointestinal issues dating back to infancy or adolescence. Patients often navigate the medical system for several years before receiving a diagnosis of MALS, with one study reporting a median duration of 5 years before MALS was finally identified [19]. During this time, patients undergo multiple diagnostic studies, including CT, MRI, ultrasound, endoscopy, colonoscopy, and often even cholecystectomy, all of which typically yield normal results. The absence of obviously detectable abnormalities on these routine tests complicates the diagnostic process. It may lead to misdiagnosis, such as somatic symptom disorder, or adjunct diagnoses, like psychiatric or eating disorders. Most patients frequent the emergency department for acute symptom management, precipitating repeat studies and increasing frustration and costs.

Interestingly, the onset of symptoms can sometimes be rapid, particularly following immune-mediated inflammation, such as in the COVID-19 infection. Studies have suggested a potential link between long-term COVID and the reactivity of autonomic nerves, which may trigger or exacerbate symptoms of MALS [20]. Additionally, physical stress, particularly in athletes, has been implicated as a potential trigger for rapid symptom onset in some individuals.

A notable aspect of MALS presentation is the presence of feeding tubes or a history of total parenteral nutrition (TPN) in some patients, including pediatric patients, highlighting the severity of their symptoms and the challenges they face in maintaining adequate nutrition. The association between MALS and immune-mediated inflammation further underscores the complexity of the syndrome and its potential triggers.

Pediatric patients present distinct challenges and considerations. Pediatric MALS patients often manifest with chronic functional abdominal pain (CFAP) [21], posing diagnostic complexities. Our review of existing studies found a prevalence of MALS among pediatric patients in their mid-to-late teens, particularly females [18]. Diagnostic modalities such as duplex ultrasound and computed tomography play pivotal roles in confirming MALS diagnosis in this population. Emphasizing pediatric-specific presentation nuances is crucial for clinicians to promptly recognize and address MALS in young patients, ensuring optimal care delivery and improved patient outcomes.

Most patients with MALS seek medical attention through nontraditional channels, such as self-referral or social media support. This occurs for a variety of reasons, including general ignorance of MALS within the medical community, overall suspicion and controversy as to the etiology of MALS (vascular vs. neurogenic), and the lack of routine exposure in clinical practice to MALS. There are robust support groups on all social media platforms, where patients and their support people find access to information and community. There is a significant risk of misinformation within these groups, but, in fairness, the questions and guidance found therein often result in successful self-advocacy and diagnosis. The frustration and desperation experienced by individuals struggling with undiagnosed or poorly managed symptoms is real and must be acknowledged. In contrast, referrals from specialists, such as gastroenterologists, cardiologists, vascular surgeons, or primary care physicians, are less common, reflecting a lack of awareness among healthcare providers regarding the diverse clinical presentations of MALS.

Differential Diagnosis of Median Arcuate Ligament Syndrome (MALS)

Diagnosing MALS presents a formidable challenge due to its ambiguous symptomatology and the necessity to rule out various alternative diagnoses. The symptoms of MALS, including epigastric abdominal pain, nausea, and weight loss, are nonspecific and overlap with a multitude of other conditions, complicating the diagnostic process. Consequently, MALS is often diagnosed by exclusion [4], requiring healthcare providers to meticulously eliminate alternative etiologies before arriving at a definitive diagnosis. This process involves assessing and addressing gallbladder disease, gastroesophageal reflux disease (GERD), ulcers, gastroparesis, irritable bowel syndrome (IBS), dysmotility, chronic constipation, mental health disorders, eating disorders, conversion disorders, and musculoskeletal injuries. On the other hand, aside from peptic ulcer disease and perhaps gastroparesis, very few conditions cause debilitating epigastric abdominal pain from all types of foods and liquids, leading to sitophobia and profound weight loss, which is nearly always the case amongst MALS patients.

MALS shares some clinical similarities with other nonocclusive compression disorders, such as superior mesenteric artery syndrome (SMAS), nutcracker syndrome [22], and May-Thurner's syndrome. Sometimes, patients with these syndromes present with symptoms resembling those of MALS, necessitating careful consideration and differentiation to arrive at an accurate diagnosis [1]. Distinguishing between these conditions requires a comprehensive evaluation of clinical symptoms, imaging studies, and specialized diagnostic tests, adding complexity to the diagnostic process.

Finally, there are a host of concomitant diseases that often correlate with MALS and other anatomic nonocclusive compressions, including Ehler's-Danlos syndrome (EDS), mast cell activation syndrome (MCAS), postural orthostatic tachycardia syndrome (POTS), etc. It is common for patients with MALS and these other syndromes to have a cross-contaminated etiology of symptoms and exacerbations.

Navigating the extensive list of potential differential diagnoses demands a systematic and thorough approach. Clinicians must meticulously evaluate the patient's medical history, perform a detailed physical examination, and employ a variety of diagnostic modalities to arrive at an accurate diagnosis. Collaboration among multiple medical specialties, including gastroenterology, surgery, radiology, and psychiatry, is often imperative to ensure a comprehensive evaluation and effective management of the condition.

Conclusion

Median arcuate ligament syndrome (MALS) presents a diagnostic challenge characterized by its nonspecific symptoms and the need to exclude numerous alternative diagnoses. The diagnostic journey often involves a process of elimination, ruling out various conditions with overlapping symptoms. Additionally, the resemblance of MALS to other compression disorders further complicates the differential diagnosis, requiring careful consideration and differentiation. A multidisciplinary approach integrating clinical expertise from multiple specialties is essential to navigate the complexities of MALS diagnosis and ensure optimal patient care. By refining diagnostic strategies and raising awareness among healthcare providers, we can enhance the recognition and management of MALS, ultimately improving patient outcomes and quality of life.

References

1. Weber JM, et al. Median arcuate ligament syndrome is not a vascular disease. Ann Vasc Surg. 2016;30:22–7.
2. Bech FR. Celiac artery compression syndromes. Surg Clin N Am. 1997;77(2):409–24.
3. Dunbar JD, et al. Compression of the celiac trunk and abdominal angina: preliminary report of 15 cases. Am J Roentgenol. 1965;95(3):731–44.
4. Kim EN, et al. Median arcuate ligament syndrome—review of this rare disease. JAMA Surg. 2016;151(5):471–7.
5. Cusati D, Noel A, Gloviczki P. Median arcuate ligament syndrome: a 20-year experience of surgical treatment. In: 60th annual meeting of the Society for Vascular Surgery. 2006.
6. Goodall R, et al. Median arcuate ligament syndrome. J Vasc Surg. 2020;71(6):2170–6.
7. Ho KKF, et al. Outcome predictors in median arcuate ligament syndrome. J Vasc Surg. 2017;65(6):1745–52.
8. Duffy AJ, et al. Management of median arcuate ligament syndrome: a new paradigm. Ann Vasc Surg. 2009;23(6):778–84.
9. Gloviczki P, Duncan AA. Treatment of celiac artery compression syndrome: does it really exist? Perspect Vasc Surg Endovasc Ther. 2007;19(3):259–63.
10. Tarbell SE, et al. Relationship among nausea, anxiety, and orthostatic symptoms in pediatric patients with chronic unexplained nausea. Exp Brain Res. 2014;232:2645–50.
11. Abdallah H, et al. Median arcuate ligament syndrome presenting as POTS. Autonomic Neurosci Basic Clin. 2015;192:123.
12. Huynh DT, et al. Median arcuate ligament syndrome and its associated conditions. Am Surg. 2019;85(10):1162–5.
13. Selvaraj BJ, et al. Celiac plexus block as a diagnostic tool in suspected pediatric median arcuate ligament syndrome. Local Reg Anesth. 2019;12:15–8.
14. Sun Z, et al. Celiac plexus block as a predictor of surgical outcome for sympathetically mediated abdominal pain in a case of suspected median arcuate ligament syndrome: a case report. A A Pract. 2018;11(3):76–8.
15. Duncan AA. Median arcuate ligament syndrome. Curr Treat Options Cardiovasc Med. 2008;10(2):112–6.
16. Skelly CL, et al. The impact of psychiatric comorbidities on patient-reported surgical outcomes in adults treated for the median arcuate ligament syndrome. J Vasc Surg. 2018;68(5):1414–21.

17. Feldman EC, et al. Psychiatric comorbidities of median arcuate ligament syndrome: Indications for intervention across the lifespan. Curr Res Psychiatry. 2021;1(2):17–9.
18. Mak GZ, et al. Pediatric chronic abdominal pain and median arcuate ligament syndrome: a review and psychosocial comparison. Pediatr Ann. 2016;45(7):e257–64.
19. Ruff GM. Evaluating initial misdiagnosis in patients with median arcuate ligament syndrome and superior mesenteric artery syndrome: a prospective analysis.
20. Dani M, et al. Autonomic dysfunction in 'long COVID': rationale, physiology and management strategies. Clin Med. 2021;21(1):e63–7.
21. Mak GZ, et al. Median arcuate ligament syndrome in the pediatric population. J Pediatr Surg. 2013;48(11):2261–70.
22. Farina R, et al. A man with the rare simultaneous combination of three abdominal vascular compression syndromes: median arcuate ligament syndrome, superior mesenteric artery syndrome, and nutcracker syndrome. Radiol Case Rep. 2021;16(6):1264–70.

Chapter 5
Diagnostic Testing (Duplex Ultrasound, CTA, MRA, Visceral Angiography, Celiac Ganglion Nerve Block) for Median Arcuate Ligament Syndrome

Katherine Fay and Ankit D. Patel

Introduction

Median arcuate ligament syndrome (MALS) is a rare clinical syndrome. Guidelines for imaging diagnostics primarily come from the European Society for Vascular Surgery (ESVS) clinical practice guidelines for chronic mesenteric ischemia [1]. Although this is generally applied to multivessel stenosis in the setting of atherosclerosis and is of limited applicability, MALS is considered the most common cause of single-vessel mesenteric ischemia [2]. Regardless of the imaging modality, findings suggestive of celiac trunk compression include focal narrowing of the superior aspect of the proximal celiac trunk, post-stenotic dilation, and/or evidence of collateral formation in the absence of atherosclerosis or other pathology. The inspiratory cycle phase also plays a large role in the degree of narrowing of the celiac trunk seen on duplex ultrasonography (US), where the degree of stenosis is exacerbated during the end of the expiratory phase as the celiac artery tracks cephalad, leading to external compression and increased flow velocities [3]. For this reason, it is recommended that imaging measurements are acquired during the end-inspiratory phase to reduce false-positive rates. Here, we describe the most commonly used imaging modalities to aid in this rare diagnosis.

K. Fay (✉) · A. D. Patel
School of Medicine, Emory University, Atlanta, GA, USA
e-mail: Kat.fay@emory.edu

D. Shouhed et al. (eds.), *Median Arcuate Ligament Syndrome*,
https://doi.org/10.1007/978-3-031-80740-4_5

Duplex Ultrasonography

Duplex ultrasonography (US) is a noninvasive imaging tool that assesses systolic peak velocities of the celiac artery during the inspiratory and expiratory phases of respiration and is generally considered to be the first-line imaging study [1]. Compared to other imaging modalities, US carries an advantage in terms of cost-effectiveness and in minimizing patient radiation exposure; however, it is operator-dependent and affected by body habitus, as well as overlying bowel gas patterns, which can decrease accuracy.

Both flow velocities and angulation of the celiac artery are evaluated when diagnosing MALS with US. The peak systolic flow velocities (PSVs) of the celiac artery in healthy patients range from 67 to 187 cm/s (mean 148 cm/s) [4]. A retrospective cohort study evaluated the effectiveness of duplex ultrasonography in patients who were ultimately diagnosed with MALS and found that the combination of a maximum expiratory volume of >350 cm/s and a celiac artery deflection angle (DA) >50° had a high probability of accurate diagnosis [5]. Of 364 patients with suspected celiac trunk pathology who underwent US of the celiac trunk, six were clinically diagnosed with MALS. Compared to the asymptomatic control group, there were significant differences in expiratory PSVs in the MALS patients (mean PSV, 425 ± 130.1 cm/s vs mean PSV, 209.9 ± 80.1 cm/s; two-tailed Mann-Whitney U, $p = 0.001$). Additionally, all diagnosed patients demonstrated a celiac artery trunk DA of >50°. The authors concluded that the combination of these two factors had an 83% sensitivity, 100% specificity, and 100% positive predictive value for diagnosis of MALS.

Computed Tomography and Magnetic Resonance Angiography

Computed tomography angiography (CTA) has long-standing been the imaging modality of choice given its ability to produce three-dimensional images, provide multiple angles of the celiac trunk take off to allow for evaluation of angulation, and allow for the possibility of evaluating other differential diagnoses compared to US. Limitations include the necessity of high loads of contrast dye, which can be problematic for patients with underlying renal dysfunction.

Evidence of focal narrowing in the proximal celiac axis with a "hooked" appearance is said to be characteristic and distinct from atherosclerotic disease or other pathology that can cause narrowing [6] (Fig. 5.1a). However, the degree of stenosis does not appear to correlate with the presence of or the severity of symptoms. Several studies have found that despite having radiographic findings suggestive of MALS, only a small percentage of patients endorse clinical symptoms consistent with the disease. Petnys et al. performed a retrospective study of 344 patients undergoing CTA for live organ donation and found that 3.4% of asymptomatic patients

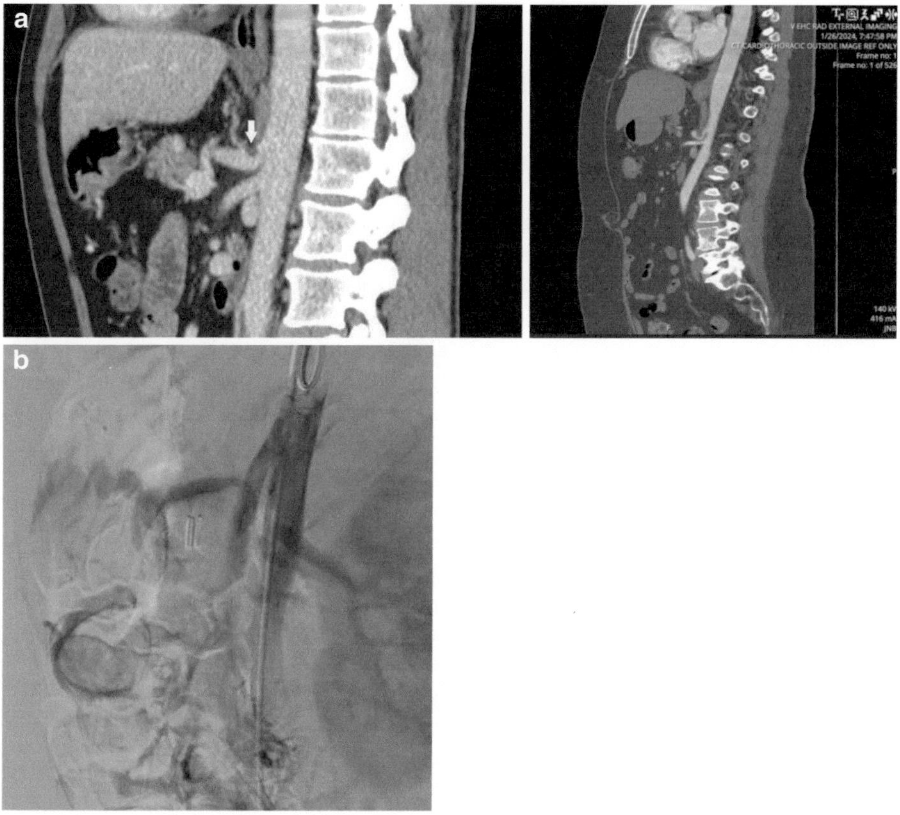

Fig. 5.1 Radiographic imaging suggestive of median arcuate ligament syndrome. (**a**) Computed tomography with arteriogram demonstrating a "classic hook" appearance of compressed celiac artery plexus. (**b**) Selective angiography demonstrating a narrowing of celiac artery takeoff

demonstrated a celiac artery compression of >50% [7]. Another retrospective study reviewed 744 CTAs obtained for various indications and found that 21 patients (2.8%) had evidence of celiac artery compression; however, only 3 of the 21 patients (14%) reported symptoms [8]. Finally, a retrospective observation study by Baskan et al. evaluated over 1000 patients with CTA and demonstrated the finding of >50% celiac artery stenosis only correlated to clinical symptoms in roughly 12% of patients (1 in 8) [9]. Given this, the authors elucidated on other findings that are suggestive but not diagnostic including post-stenotic dilation of the celiac artery, which is better appreciated on CTA compared to US. This also suggests that celiac axis neurogenic dysfunction may play a role in the clinical presentation of MALS as opposed to symptoms being purely from celiac artery compression [10].

Magnetic resonance angiography (MRA) has the advantage of not utilizing ionizing radiation which may be a safer option in pediatric patients, patients with renal disease, or patients with a contrast allergy. This imaging modality provides similar findings as CTA.

Visceral Angiography

The addition of arterial visceral angiography also allows for the detection of collateral development in the setting of celiac artery stenosis (Fig. 5.1b). Arazińska et al. noted a significant correlation between the degree of isolated celiac artery stenosis and the development of mesenteric collaterals (Spearman's coefficient 0.275, $p < 0.006$), suggesting that a higher degree of stenosis may result in a higher ischemia risk and thus the development of alternative vascular pathways to mitigate this [11]. These findings are pertinent in that some studies have suggested that the development of mesenteric collateralization in patients with MALS may portend a less favorable outcome following surgical intervention. Van Peterson et al. performed a single-institution retrospective review of 129 patients who underwent median arcuate ligament release between 2002 and 2013 [12]. Preoperative angiography was used to determine the degree of collateralization; a favorable postoperative outcome was determined by <50% restenosis rate on inspiratory/expiratory duplex US and clinical resolution of symptoms or sustained reduction in symptoms. The study found that the degree of clinical success was inversely related to the number of collaterals developed, where only 52% of patients with grade 2 collaterals (defined as at least vessel visible on nonselective angiography) had symptom resolution compared to 81% of patients with grade 0 collaterals (defined as no visible collaterals) [12].

Gastric Exercise Tonometry

Gastric exercise tonometry is an additional imaging adjunct that can diagnose mesenteric ischemia as related to MALS diagnosis. A catheter is placed into the gastric lumen and intramucosal and intraluminal $PaCO_2$ values are assessed prior to, during, and after submaximal exercise. Results consistent with pathologic ischemia include an increase in gastric $PaCO_2$ after exercise with a change greater than 0.8 kPa and an arterial lactate less than 72 mg/dL [13, 14]. Mensink et al. performed a retrospective study looking at 43 patients with evidence of celiac artery compression on selective angiography who subsequently underwent gastric exercise tonometry [15]. Twenty-nine (67%) of these patients had evidence of ischemia; all patients subsequently underwent surgical intervention with 22 patients undergoing median arcuate ligament release (5 patients underwent venous patching; two underwent autologous bypass). At follow-up, 24 (83%) of 29 patients were asymptomatic; of the 16 asymptomatic patients who underwent post-intervention gastric tonometry, all 16 demonstrated a statistically significant decrease in maximal $PaCO_2$ gradient (1.5 ± 0.4 to 0.7 ± 0.3 post-intervention, $p < 0.0001$).

Celiac Ganglion Nerve Block

In addition to focal narrowing of the celiac artery, the pathophysiology of MALS has thought to include compression of the celiac ganglia plexus resulting in a neurogenic contribution to the presentation of abdominal pain [16, 17]. This theory is reinforced by several studies that have demonstrated that a celiac plexus block may be a strong indicator of success following surgical intervention for MALS which includes celiac ganglionectomy [18]. A celiac plexus block can be performed in a variety of different ways with most utilizing fluoroscopy for visualization. Approach techniques include retrocrural, antecrural, transaortic, and an anterior approach. Additionally, the celiac plexus can be targeted through an endoscopically guided approach, but this is dependent upon having access to a trained gastroenterologist and the necessary equipment, which may not be available at all medical facilities. Each fluoroscopic technique has its own associated risks and benefits with no studies to indicate superiority of one approach compared to the other; however, the literature has noted some shortcomings. Due to is location, a retrocrural approach targets the splanchnic nerves supplying the celiac plexus, rather than the celiac plexus itself which may alter outcomes. Additionally, an antecrural approach has a larger target area necessitating a larger volume of anesthetic injected in order to achieve the same benefit. The transaortic and anterior approaches are associated with an increased risk of retroperitoneal hemorrhage and damage to nearby visceral organs, respectively.

Conclusion

Multiple imaging modalities are available to aid in the diagnosis of MALS. However, given the nonspecific imaging characteristics, MALS should remain a clinical diagnosis of exclusion, and imaging findings should be supported by symptom presentation. Radiographic findings are an important adjunct but may not be the defining element of diagnosis.

References

1. Björck M, Koelemay M, Acosta S, et al. Management of the diseases of mesenteric arteries and veins: clinical practice guidelines of the European Society of Vascular Surgery (ESVS). Eur J Vasc Endovasc Surg. 2017;53(4):460–510.
2. Goodall R, Langridge B, Onida S, Ellis M, Lane T, Davies AH. Median arcuate ligament syndrome. J Vasc Surg. 2020;71(6):2170–6.
3. Skeik N, Cooper LT, Duncan AA, Jabr FI. Median arcuate ligament syndrome: a nonvascular, vascular diagnosis. Vasc Endovasc Surg. 2011;45(5):433–7.
4. AbuRahma AF, et al. Mesenteric/celiac duplex ultrasound interpretation criteria revisited. J Vasc Surg. 2012;55(2):428–36.

5. Gruber H, Loizides A, Peer S, Gruber I. Ultrasound of the median arcuate ligament syndrome: a new approach to diagnosis. Med Ultrason. 2012;14(1):5–9.
6. Horton KM, Talamini MA, Fishman EK. Median arcuate ligament syndrome: evaluation with CT angiography. Radiographics. 2005;25(5):1177–82.
7. Petnys A, Puech-Leão P, Zerati AE, Ritti-Dias RM, Nahas WC, Neto ED, et al. Prevalence of signs of celiac axis compression by the median arcuate ligament on computed tomography angiography in asymptomatic patients. J Vasc Surg. 2018;68:1782–7.
8. Gümüs H, Gümüs M, Tekbas G, Önder H, Ekici F, Cetinçakmak MG, et al. Clinical and multidetector computed tomography findings of patients with median arcuate ligament syndrome. Clin Imaging. 2012;36:522–5.
9. Baskan O, Kaya E, Gungoren FZ, Erol C. Compression of the celiac artery by the median arcuate ligament: multidetector computed tomography findings and characteristics. Can Assoc Radiol J. 2015;66(3):272–6.
10. Chaum M, et al. Clinico-pathologic findings in patients with median arcuate ligament syndrome (celiac artery compression syndrome). Ann Diagn Pathol. 2021;52:151732.
11. Arazińska A, Polguj M, Wojciechowski A, Trębiński Ł, Stefańczyk L. Median arcuate ligament syndrome: predictor of ischemic complications? Clin Anat. 2016;29(8):1025–30.
12. van Petersen AS, Kolkman JJ, Gerrits DG, et al. Clinical significance of mesenteric arterial collateral circulation in patients with celiac artery compression syndrome. J Vasc Surg. 2017;65(5):1366–74.
13. Kolkman JJ, Otte JA, Groeneveld AB. Gastrointestinal luminal PCO_2 tonometry: an update on physiology, methodology and clinical applications. Br J Anaesth. 2000;84(1):74–86.
14. Groeneveld AB, Kolkman JJ. Splanchnic tonometry: a review of physiology, methodology, and clinical applications. J Crit Care. 1994;9(3):198–210.
15. Mensink PB, van Petersen AS, Kolkman JJ, Otte JA, Huisman AB, Geelkerken RH. Gastric exercise tonometry: the key investigation in patients with suspected celiac artery compression syndrome. J Vasc Surg. 2006;44(2):277–81.
16. Suzuki K, Kashimura H, Sato M, Hassan M, Yokota H, Nakahara A, et al. Pancreaticoduodenal artery aneurysms associated with celiac axis stenosis due to compression by median arcuate ligament and celiac plexus. J Gastroenterol. 1998;33:434–8.
17. Balaban DH, Chen J, Lin Z, Tribble CG, McCallum RW. Median arcuate ligament syndrome: a possible cause of idiopathic gastroparesis. Am J Gastroenterol. 1997;92(3):519–23.
18. Sun Z, Fritz DA, Turner S, et al. Celiac plexus block as a predictor of surgical outcome for sympathetically mediated abdominal pain in a case of suspected median arcuate ligament syndrome: a case report. A A Pract. 2018;11(3):76–8.
19. Titton RL, Lucey BC, Gervais DA, Boland GW, Mueller PR. Celiac plexus block: a palliative tool underused by radiologists. Am J Roentgenol. 2002;179(3):633–6.

Chapter 6
Conditions Associated with Median Arcuate Ligament Syndrome: POTS, MCAS, EDS

Jamie DeCicco, Jessica Johnson, and Robert Wilson

Mast Cell Activation Syndrome (MCAS

Mast cell activation syndrome (MCAS) was first utilized in the late 1980s to describe variants of systemic mastocytosis. The term mast cell disease (MCD) encompasses a range of disorders, including systemic mastocytosis (SM), cutaneous mastocytosis (CM), mast cell activation syndrome (MCAS), and hereditary alpha tryptasemia (HaT) [1]. While most of these disorders involve an abnormal increase in mast cells in tissues, MCAS does not involve mast cell proliferation [2, 3]. Instead, individuals suffering from MCAS have mast cells that degranulate at a lower threshold and in response to environmental/chemical triggers that are benign. The term MCAS has become more widely used in recent years and describes those suffering from a host of symptoms not limited to the gastrointestinal (nausea, vomiting, diarrhea, abdominal pain, malabsorption, gastroesophageal reflux), dermatological (flushing, urticaria, rashes), cardiovascular (blood pressure dysregulation, tachycardia, chest pain), and neurological systems (dizziness, migraines, brain fog, peripheral neuropathy) [3].

Mast cells are concentrated in tissues exposed to the environment and play a critical role in the innate and adaptive immune systems. Most commonly

J. DeCicco (✉) · J. Johnson
Cleveland Clinic Lerner College of Medicine of Case Western Reserve University, Cleveland, OH, USA

R. Wilson
Cleveland Clinic Lerner College of Medicine of Case Western Reserve University, Cleveland, OH, USA

Department of Neurology, Neuromuscular Center, Cleveland Clinic, Cleveland, OH, USA
e-mail: wilsonr3@ccf.org

D. Shouhed et al. (eds.), *Median Arcuate Ligament Syndrome*,
https://doi.org/10.1007/978-3-031-80740-4_6

understood to play a role in allergic disease, mast cells can be activated by both IgE-dependent and IgE-independent mechanisms. Once activated, mast cells degranulate and release multiple molecules, including tryptase, histamine, prostaglandin, leukotrienes, heparin, proteases, and TNFa [3]. Specifically in the gut, the mediators most commonly associated with GI manifestations are tryptase and chymase. It is this process of degranulation that leads to the host of clinical signs/symptoms associated with MCAS.

Serum tryptase is the most specific marker of mast cell activation and is one of the many molecules released during mast cell degranulation [4]. A normal tryptase level is considered 5 ng/ml or below. A level greater than 11.4 ng/ml is elevated, and any level above 20 ng/ml should prompt a diagnostic rule out of systemic mastocytosis. Tryptase levels peak approximately 1 to 4 hours after a mast cell degranulation event. An elevation of 20% of baseline serum tryptase plus 2 ng/ml is recognized as a mast cell activation episode. Up to 6% of the general population have elevated basal serum tryptase levels, for reasons that have not been elucidated [5]. Some of these individuals with inherited elevated tryptase levels present with multisystem complaints similar to the MCAS symptoms described previously. Recent studies have shown that the elevated tryptase levels in some individuals arise out of a germline duplication and triplication in the TPSAB1 gene, which encodes for alpha-tryptase [5]. The result is an elevated basal tryptase level. Interestingly, a dose effect is present. Individuals with 3 copies of the alpha-tryptase gene had higher basal serum levels of tryptase and reported more symptoms when compared to those with two copies of the alpha-tryptase gene in a study of 96 subjects from 35 affected families [5].

Within the 35 affected families with elevated basal tryptase levels, symptoms associated with MCAS were seen at much higher rates than in the general population [5]. Specifically, gastrointestinal dysmotility, manifesting most frequently as irritable bowel syndrome or chronic gastroesophageal reflux, was seen at rates 3–5× higher than the general population. Connective tissue abnormalities, such as joint hypermobility, were seen in 28% of individuals in this cohort. Those with connective tissue abnormalities also reported high rates of chronic arthralgia (45%) and headache (47%). Skin complaints were also frequent with cutaneous flushing and pruritus impacting 51% of the cohort. These symptoms reported appear to be inherited in a dominant pattern and have associations with joint hypermobility syndromes, such as Ehlers-Danlos. The authors of this study propose that the association between elevated tryptase levels and the multisystem disorders seen could arise out of activation of the protease-activated receptor 2 dependent pathways (PAR2) or involve coinheritance of another functional genetic variant [5].

Other studies have more specifically looked at the impact of elevated tryptase on the GI tract. More specifically, one study compared duodenal biopsies in those with hereditary alpha-tryptasemia (HaT), a terminology used to describe those with triplication of the alpha-tryptase encoding sequence, to those with MCAS, with no tryptase elevation, to controls [6]. Those with HaT had increased mast cells in the duodenum compared to the other two groups. More specifically, the HaT group had a median mast cell number of 30 (IQR 20.0–40.0) compared to the MCAS group, with no tryptase elevation, which had a median 15.0 (IQR 5.0–20.0, $p = 0.013$). The control group similarly had a median of 15 (IQR 13.8–20.0, $p = 0.004$). Thus, these results suggest that increased small intestinal mast cells could play a role in the GI symptoms seen in HaT and that tryptase levels could play a role in the mast cell recruitment and resultant symptoms seen in MCAS.

Mast cells could play a role in multiple gastrointestinal (GI) pathologies. One study hypothesized that postoperative ileus could have a mast cell component, where bowel manipulation leads to increased mast cells in the bowel wall and results in inflammation; this in turn results in the motility disturbances seen in postoperative gastroparesis and ileus [7]. Additionally, the authors cite evidence for bidirectional communication between mast cells and neurons in the GI tract, in which mast cell mediators activate nerves, which in turn release neurotransmitters that enhance mast cell activity, all together creating a positive feedback loop. Such a phenomenon has been additionally identified in irritable bowel syndrome (IBS), with studies highlighting that mast cells activate nearby neurons and may be associated with the pain seen in IBS [8]. Additionally, multiple studies have shown that symptoms of IBS correlate to the number of intestinal mast cells and the level of mediators, such as tryptase, histamine, and serotonin [9]. Interestingly, one study looking at specimens from those undergoing surgery for slow transit constipation showed an increase in colonic mast cells in those with constipation when compared to healthy controls [10]. The authors utilized immunohistochemistry for tryptase and CD117 as proxies for mast cell presence. The authors hypothesize that the increased mast cells could have been an attempt to repair the damaged neuro-enteric system. Such results could be relevant to the MALS population who present with high rates of MCAS, alongside constipation [10].

MCAS is seen at high rates in the MALS population. In one study looking at over 250 individuals with multiple compression syndromes, the authors state that many of these patients had MCAS [11]. Another study of 60 patients with MALS, reported that 9 (15%) of the individuals had a concomitant diagnosis of MCAS [12]. In a survey study of 242 patients who self-reported a MALS diagnosis, 22.6% reported a diagnosis of MCAS [13]. In another cohort study of 20 MALS patients, the authors highlight that a diagnosis of MCAS (7/20) significantly correlated with persistent MALS symptoms after surgical treatment (5/7, $p = 0.04$) [14]. The authors hypothesize that because there are overlapping GI symptoms in MALS and MCAS, some of the individuals' GI complaints arose out of MCAS instead of MALS and thus surgical interventions did not prove useful clinically.

Symptoms of MCAS that can overlap with MALS include nausea with vomiting, crampy abdominal pain, and altered bowel habits [14]. Those with MCAS present with fluctuating symptoms and identifying unique triggers can be challenging. As such, many may have negative GI and endoscopic findings, which could then be interpreted as MALS, when in reality the symptoms may arise out of a sole MCAS or mixed MCAS/MALS picture [14].

Identifying MALS patients with concomitant MCAS can be challenging. One initial screening question suggested by other authors is to inquire about a history of multiple allergies [14]. If positive, further MCAS screening tools could be considered. There is controversy around the diagnosis of MCAS, with broader inclusion criteria encompassing up to 17% of the general population [15]. Some of the current consensus criteria recognized for diagnosing MCAS include clinical signs of mast cell activation involving two or more organ systems, an elevated serum tryptase level (baseline +20%), and/or symptoms that respond to mast cell stabilizing agents and/or mast cell blockers [16]. However, these tests can be challenging to execute and interpret. Thus, at a minimum utilizing screening tools for symptoms could be considered if suspicion for MCAS is high. Additionally, MCAS is traditionally handled by allergists, thus having these patients seen and worked up by an allergist should be considered if suspicion for MCAS is high.

Ehlers-Danlos Syndrome (EDS)

Ehlers-Danlos syndrome (EDS) is a term used to describe heritable connective tissue disorders, which present with symptoms of joint hypermobility, skin hyperextensibility, and tissue fragility. Multiple genetic mutations in collagen-encoding genes or enzymes have been associated with EDS and the classification has evolved into multiple different subtypes as a result. The latest 2017 International Classification of EDS proposed the definite diagnosis of EDS requires molecular confirmation of a causative genetic variant, with the exception of the hypermobile type of EDS (hEDS) [17]. The genetic basis for hEDS is still unknown, though the inheritance pattern appears to be autosomal dominant. hEDS will be the focus of this chapter.

hEDS is the most common type of EDS [18]. Defining an exact prevalence for hEDS has proved challenging because of the lack of a clear diagnostic test for hEDS. Additionally, hEDS presents as a spectrum of severity so patients may go undiagnosed for many years. Generalized joint hypermobility, defined as impacting four or more joints, has a reported prevalence between 12–28% of the population [18]. However, many individuals have joint hypermobility with no clinical effects, while others present with symptom severity and comorbidities similar to hEDS. One study in Wales reported a prevalence of hEDS and hypermobility spectrum disorder (HSD) as 1 in 500, with 70% of these individuals identifying as female [19]. Females make up an unusually large proportion of those with hEDS, despite a suspected autosomal dominant inheritance pattern. Gender differences, such as muscle mass and ligament stability, could explain some of these clinical differences. The sexual dimorphism in hEDS is currently under investigation by multiple research groups [20].

hEDS presents with a progression of disease [18]. The first phase presents in childhood with ligament laxity as well as frequent dislocations and subluxations, with no/minimum complaints of pain. The second phase, called the "pain phase," arises when individuals are in their 20s and joint hypermobility may begin to decrease, but pain begins to worsen. The third phase, called the "stiffness phase," arises later in life and results in limited joint mobility and chronic pain.

Diagnosing hEDS requires the presence of 3 criteria, according to the most recent 2017 International Classification of EDS. A key part of the diagnostic criteria is the Beighton Scoring System [21]. This is a nine-point scale that can be done in the office as a measure of joint hypermobility. A higher score indicates increased joint hypermobility. While the Beighton score cannot diagnose hEDS, it can provide guidance on future testing. An abbreviated version of the diagnostic criteria for hEDS is below [22]. For more information one can access the International Consortium on Ehlers-Danlos Syndrome and Related Disorders and the Ehlers-Danlos website for more extensive questions and printouts for patients.

Criteria 1—one of the following:

- Beighton score ≥6 in prepubertal children and adolescents
- Beighton score ≥5 in pubertal men and woman to age 50
- Beighton score ≥4 in both men and women over the age of 50

Criteria 2—Two or more of the following features (A, B, or C) must be present:

- Feature A
  - Soft/velvety skin or skin hyperextensibility
  - Atrophic scarring and/or unexplained striae without a history of significant loss of body fat
  - Pelvic floor, rectal, and or uterine prolapse in children, men, or nulliparous woman without a history of morbid obesity
  - Dental crowding and high or narrow palate
  - Mitral valve prolapse
  - Aortic root dilatation
- Feature B
  - Positive family history
- Feature C
  - Musculoskeletal pain in two or more limbs, recurring daily for at least 3 months
  - Chronic, widespread pain for ≥3 months
  - Recurrent joint dislocations and/or joint instability

If all three criteria are not met, individuals may alternatively be diagnosed with hypermobility spectrum disorder (HSD) [18]. However, it is important to recognize that individuals with HSD can present with similar severity of symptoms as hEDS, as well as similar comorbidities [20]. Additionally, over time, individuals can move from the HSD category to hEDS. Thus, while diagnosing these patients is critical, the actual label of their disease may not correlate to symptom severity and management.

GI complaints are commonly reported among those with hEDS. Specifically, the most commonly reported symptoms are gastroesophageal reflux disease (GERD) (79.3%), irritable bowel syndrome (48%), and motility issues (48%) [18]. A survey done at the Mayo Clinic of 687 EDS patients, most of whom had hEDS, showed that 56% reported some GI manifestation and 28.3% who underwent colonic transit studies had an abnormally fast or slow transit [23]. Of this group, the most common GI symptoms were abdominal pain (56.1%), nausea (42.3%), constipation (38.6%), heartburn (37.6%), and IBS-like symptoms (27.5%) [24]. Another study that looked at GI symptoms in hEDS patients, compared to age and sex-matched controls, showed much higher rates of reported GI symptoms (37% versus 11%) [24]. Hyperextensibility of the GI tract is one proposed mechanism of the high rates of functional GI disorders seen in hEDS [25]. Another potential mechanism is the high rate of mast cell disorder seen in those with hEDS. Studies have reported a prevalence of mast cell disorder as high as 66% amongst those with hEDS.

There is a high prevalence of hEDS among MALS patients. A 60 person cohort of MALS patients showed a prevalence of hEDS of 12.5% and another study of 11 patients showed a rate of 11.8% [12]. An additional study of 11 MALS patients had two affected by hEDS (18.2%) [26]. In a survey study of 242 patients who self-reported a MALS diagnosis, 31.7% reported a diagnosis of EDS [13]. These rates are much higher than the general population, even with the understanding that hEDS is underdiagnosed.

No clear relationship between hEDS and MALS has been presented in the literature. One proposed hypothesis involves the anatomical changes that arise in puberty in females versus males [27]. Specifically, during puberty the female pelvis becomes wider and deeper, which causes positional changes in the lumbar spine. The increased lordosis of the lumbar spine leads to compression of the anatomic structures that lie in front of the spine. With loss of weight, the lordosis appears to increase, worsening the compression syndromes. This hypothesis is further supported by the fact that hEDS and MALS predominantly occur in females. Additionally, in hEDS, there is increased mobility of all joints. As such, scoliosis frequently occurs in hEDS, with a reported prevalence of 52% [28]. Thus, the increased rates of scoliosis seen in hEDS, alongside generalized spinal mobility, could further explain the association of hEDS not only with MALS but also with multiple compression syndromes. Studies have shown that hEDS is especially associated with patients who present with three or more compression syndromes (Nutcracker syndrome, May-Thurner syndrome, superior mesenteric artery syndrome) [11]. In particular, these patients have poor outcomes when just treated for one compression syndrome, and in fact, the other compression syndromes usually worsen after a single correction. Importantly, correction of all the vascular compression syndromes leads to improvement or resolution of symptoms.

Functional rib pain syndromes should also be considered in patients with hEDS and symptoms of vascular compression syndromes. In slipped rib syndrome, one or more of the 8th-10th ribs can become abnormally mobile and sublux internally, irritating the diaphragm and causing upper abdominal pain [29]. Patients may experience visceral disturbances such as tachycardia, dyspnea, GERD, early satiety, nausea, gastroparesis, constipation, and IBS [30]. Many of these symptoms overlap with presentations in POTS and MALS, so it is important to conduct a physical exam evaluating for rib hypermobility and reproducible dermatomal pain on palpation to rule out another possible cause for patient presentation. The abnormal vertical orientation of the ribs and migration down to the pelvis due to increased thoracic joint laxity may result in rib tip syndrome with costo-iliac impingement [29, 31]. This condition, along with 12th rib syndrome and L1 syndrome, may mimic symptoms of nutcracker or May-Thurner syndrome.

Postural Orthostatic Tachycardia Syndrome (POTS)

Postural orthostatic tachycardia syndrome (POTS) is a complex chronic disorder of the autonomic nervous system characterized by an exaggerated heart rate response to standing or changing positions to an upright posture [32]. This can result in symptoms of lightheadedness, presyncope, dizziness, palpitations, and fatigue. In addition to the abnormal circulatory response to position changes, patients may also experience cognitive impairment or "brain fog," low energy, muscle exhaustion, exercise intolerance, generalized weakness, chest pain, anxiety, migraine headaches, and gastrointestinal symptoms (bloating, nausea, diarrhea, abdominal pain, etc.) [32–34]. The list below defines an abbreviated version of the consensus diagnostic criteria for POTS [34–36]. All five criteria must be met for POTS diagnosis.

1. A sustained increase in heart rate by 30 beats/min (bpm) or maximum heart rate of 120 bpm within 10 min of standing or head-up tilt.
   (a) A simple supine to standing test may be used, or a tilt table test if vital signs need to be monitored for longer periods.
   (b) For individuals aged 12–19 years old, the required HR increase is at least 40 bpm.
2. An absence of orthostatic hypotension (no sustained drop in blood pressure ≥20/10 mmHg) within 3 min of upright posture
3. Frequent symptoms of orthostatic intolerance during standing, with rapid improvement upon return to a supine position.
4. Duration of symptoms for at least 3 months
5. Absence of other conditions explaining sinus tachycardia such as medications, acute physiologic stimuli, nutrition and hydration status, or other medical conditions [34–36].

POTS is estimated to affect 1–3 million individuals in the United States [35], although the prevalence has not been properly studied and is likely even higher after the COVID-19 pandemic, as post-COVID POTS is a frequent occurrence. POTS most commonly occurs in females with a female-to-male ratio of 5:1. The majority of patients present between 15 and 25 years of age [32]. A number of possible triggers for POTS have been proposed, including immunologic stressors (such as viral syndromes), physical trauma (such as concussions or surgery), and, specific to females, menarche and pregnancy, which have been associated with disease onset [35, 37].

While the exact etiology is not well established, there are multiple potential pathophysiologic mechanisms for POTS, including but not limited to neuropathic, hypovolemic, hyperadrenergic, and immune processes. These categories are not mutually exclusive as patients may have more than one mechanism contributing to their symptoms.

The neuropathic phenotype is present in about 50% of patients and is thought to result from partial sympathetic denervation, with evidence of small fiber neuropathy (SFN) present in many patients [38]. Because small nerve fibers communicate sensory sensations and regulate the autonomic nervous system, nerve dysfunction can lead to a variety of symptoms, including pain, decreased sweating, dry eyes and mouth, orthostatic dizziness, palpitations, urinary retention, gastroparesis, constipation, hypo- or hyperhidrosis, and skin discoloration [39–41]. The COMPASS 31 survey can be a useful screening tool in determining symptom burden and if SFN is likely to play a role in a patient's case. Objectively, abnormalities on thermoregulatory sweat testing, quantitative sudomotor axon reflex testing, and unmyelinated nerve fibers on a skin biopsy may be present.

There is a high rate of POTS and orthostatic dysfunction in those with hEDS. Connective tissue abnormalities can result in sympathetic activation and a hyperadrenergic POTS phenotype. Additionally, hEDS patients have high rates of small fiber neuropathy and autonomic neuropathy [42]. In a cohort of 31 patients with hEDS, 19 (61%) were diagnosed with SFN utilizing skin biopsy [42]. The SFN was defined as a degeneration of distal nerve endings. Of those with SFN, 63% had length-dependent SFN and 32% had non-length-dependent SFN. Most had clinical complaints of pain and sensory disturbances, in line with SFN. Additionally, ten (32%) also fulfilled the criteria for POTS; of note, however, 29 (94%) had orthostatic complaints. Thus, there is a strong association between hEDS and POTS, potentially explained by sympathetic activation and SFN.

Hypovolemia is common in POTS with up to 70% of patients having a reduction in red blood cell and plasma volume [36, 37]. Normally, the renin-angiotensin-aldosterone system compensates for a deficit in blood volume by increasing angiotensin II, which stimulates aldosterone to increase renal sodium and water reabsorption. However, in POTS, there are abnormalities in the levels and responsiveness to these hormones. Angiotensin II levels are two times higher than normal, but renin and aldosterone do not respond appropriately and remain low, indicating reduced vascular and adrenal responsiveness [36, 37]. Partial renal denervation may also impair sodium and water retention as well as erythropoietin production [37]. Patients may benefit from dietary sodium, intravenous saline or albumin infusions, or desmopressin to increase blood volume [43].

Hyperadrenergic stimulation is the other most common presentation of POTS. Up to 50% of POTS patients have a hyperadrenergic phenotype, often in combination with sympathetic denervation and/or hypovolemia [36]. The hyperadrenergic phenotype may be characterized by a plasma norepinephrine ≥600 pg/mL with orthostatic tachycardia, an increase in systolic blood pressure ≥10 mmHg, or sympathetic activation with symptoms of palpitations, anxiety, and tremulousness when the patient stands [34, 36]. In POTS patients who have evidence of small fiber neuropathy and impaired cardiovascular autonomic function, sympathetic impairment may occur during deep breathing and the Valsalva maneuver [38]. Normally upon deep inspiration, preload decreases and heart rate increases. Upon expiration, the heart rate decreases. Specifically, during the Valsalva test, when the patient inspires and bares down, the diaphragm descends, blood pressure drops, and preload decreases. The baroreceptors respond by increasing the heart rate. When the patient expires and the diaphragm ascends, hemodynamics is restored with blood pressure and preload increasing and the heart rate decreasing. If there is sympathetic dysfunction, response to the Valsalva maneuver may be abnormal, where the patient cannot compensate for the change in pressure, leading to feelings of dyspnea in the setting of a low preload [44].

Those with hyperadrenergic POTS have high rates of MCAS. A subgroup of patients with POTS report episodic flushing and comorbid mast cell disease. In a study of 69 POTS patients, 42% had elevated biomarkers consistent with mast cell activation syndrome [45]. The first proposed mechanism is that sympathetic stimulation experienced in POTS induces mast cell degranulation [46]. The second is the activation of mast cells releases circulating vasodilators, including histamine and other neuropeptides, which then elicit reflex sympathetic activation [36, 46]. Flushing episodes may be triggered in these patients by exercise or simply standing, and they often have a hyperadrenergic phenotype [47]. As such, symptom presentation between MCAS and POTS overlaps, including lightheadedness, dizziness, dyspnea, diuresis, nausea, diarrhea, and headache [36]. Additionally, there could be an immune-related component underlying both conditions.

While the immune-mediated processes in POTS are not well understood, an estimated 20–50% of patients report development of POTS symptoms after a viral infection. A study conducted from 2015 to 2017 reports about 40% of patients had an acute infection prior to the onset of POTS [48]. With the COVID-19 pandemic, the incidence of POTS has been increasing, which has prompted further investigation into a possible immunological cause [35, 49]. After COVID, there is an increased risk of immune-mediated neurological events with a relatively rapid onset of autonomic dysfunction post-infection [50, 51]. Possible mechanisms for post-COVID POTS include infection and destruction of extracardiac postganglionic sympathetic nervous system neurons, invasion of the brainstem, and altered medullary function with increased sympathetic outflow, autoimmunity, hypovolemia, and deconditioning [52]. In an early case series of post-COVID POTS, many patients did not respond to traditional POTS treatments, but a few did respond to IVIG, providing further support for an immunologic role [51]. Other small studies have also shown the benefit of IVIG in POTS, and there are active clinical trials investigating its treatment value [53, 54]. Additional support for immune dysfunction in POTS includes a higher prevalence of autoimmune disorders compared to the general population, with approximately 20% of POTS patients having an autoimmune comorbidity [54]. Some of these include celiac disease [55], Hashimoto's thyroiditis, Sjogren's syndrome [56], and systemic lupus erythematosus [54]. There are also a number of autoantibodies currently under investigation found to be associated with POTS [54, 57].

Gastrointestinal function is regulated by the interplay between the autonomic and enteric nervous systems [35]. GI symptoms are common among patients with POTS and other autonomic disorders. In a study of symptom burden, POTS patients reported GI symptoms at rates 5.5 times higher than controls and autonomic failure/neuropathy patients at rates 6.7 times higher than controls on the COMPASS 31 [58]. Common symptoms include early satiety, bloating, abdominal pain, nausea, vomiting, diarrhea, and constipation [58, 59]. Patients may present with irritable bowel syndrome or dysmotility ranging from mild transit derangement to gastroparesis to complete intestinal failure [35]. In a study of 103 pediatric patients with orthostatic intolerance, antroduodenal manometry was abnormal in 81%, showing neurogenic intestinal dysmotility in 50%, "rumination" in 20%, and visceral hyperalgesia in 10% [60]. Gastric emptying studies were also done and shown to be abnormal in 28%, the majority of which were delayed indicating gastroparesis [60]. These results of 20–30% of patients having delayed gastric emptying have been found in other studies of GI dysfunction in POTS as well [59]. Patients with delayed gastric emptying often experience vomiting and more severe adrenergic dysfunction noted on autonomic testing, consistent with a hyperadrenergic phenotype [60]. Gastrointestinal symptoms can be reproduced during the tilt table test, suggesting postural changes as a trigger [60]. Other studies have shown abnormalities in GI transit in POTS patients but also have found a great percentage of patients with rapid gastric emptying (48%) in addition to delayed (18%) [61].

MALS may be responsible for GI symptoms in some POTS patients [62]. Of patients who have been diagnosed with MALS, POTS is one of the most common comorbidities. In a survey of 242 patients with MALS, 53% reported symptoms of dysautonomia [13]. Several studies comment on the co-occurrence of MALS and POTS, although it is unclear if they develop simultaneously or one before the other. While there is no well-established pathophysiologic relationship between the two conditions, autonomic dysfunction is a common underlying factor. The celiac ganglion contains sympathetic nerves, so compression of this ganglion in MALS can lead to overstimulation or aberrant signaling of the sympathetic nervous system, leading to POTS-like symptoms.

As in POTS, patients with MALS experience symptoms of autonomic dysfunction, of which GI dysmotility may be the most prominent. The celiac ganglia are the largest plexus of nerve bundles in the autonomic nervous system and receive their vascular supply from the celiac artery [63]. These ganglia innervate the digestive tract and abdominal visceral tissue, helping coordinate intestinal motility, secretion, and absorption [63]. The celiac ganglia have been increasingly recognized as contributing to the pathophysiology of MALS [64–66]. Therefore, nerve dysfunction could help explain some of the overlapping dysautonomia and GI dysmotility symptoms in MALS and POTS [67, 68]. In fact, there is emerging histopathologic evidence of neural injury and immune response in the celiac ganglia of patients with MALS [64]. Investigation of small fiber neuropathy would also be of interest in MALS patients to evaluate for any evidence of nerve denervation and similarities to neuropathic POTS. In a study of 93 patients with POTS and persistent gastrointestinal symptoms, evidence of MALS with dynamically elevated celiac artery velocities was identified in over 50% of their sample [69]. The authors report tremendous improvement in POTS symptoms for patients who elected to undergo MALS surgery [69]. Another case study had similar findings of POTS symptom resolution with neurolysis of the celiac ganglion [70]. This has also been shown in a pediatrics series in which over half of their 31-patient sample had improvement in their POTS symptoms after MALS surgery [71]. In another study of 41 patients with MALS and POTS, the hyperadrenergic phenotype was present in 65% and 58% had evidence of gastroparesis [72]. Laparoscopic MALS surgery resulted in orthostatic and GI symptom resolution and significant improvement in quality-of-life scores [72].

Immunologic and hormonal factors may be common links between POTS and MALS. Both conditions are predominantly seen in females with 5:1 female-to-male ratios, as is the case in autoimmune disease. POTS and MALS patients have a higher prevalence of autoimmune disorders compared to the general population [35, 64]. In a survey of 242 MALS patients, 37% reported also having an autoimmune condition [13]. Interestingly, many patients also report the development of MALS symptoms after a viral infection such as COVID-19, Coxsackie B, or Epstein Barr virus, which are some of the most common triggers for POTS. Studies further defining the prevalence of autoimmune disorders in MALS and which ones are most common, as well as studies quantifying the number of MALS cases preceded by a viral illness will be helpful to better understand these patterns. Future research into possible autoantibodies and treatments such as IVIG would be of interest, as these are also being investigated in POTS and MCAS.

Many patients with MALS have pain and difficulty with deep breathing. This may be due to impairment in blood flow through the celiac artery, which is exaggerated during expiration as well as pain in the median arcuate ligament of the diaphragm and celiac ganglion. In POTS, small fiber neuropathy and impaired cardiovascular autonomic function contribute to sympathetic impairment of deep breathing and abnormalities in the Valsalva maneuver. It would be of interest to assess the hemodynamics and the Valsalva response in patients with MALS and see if any abnormalities exist with their ability to compensate, possibly due to sympathetic impairment as in POTS or limited by pain.

Patients with MALS commonly have severe pain, nausea, and vomiting while eating and drinking, putting them at risk for malnutrition and dehydration. This depleted nutritional state in combination with other autonomic symptoms may limit their activity, leading to weight loss and physical deconditioning. Cardiac atrophy and hypovolemia have been proposed to contribute to orthostatic tachycardia as a physiologic response to smaller stroke volume in POTS and may also apply to MALS [73]. Therefore, nutritional optimization with potential support via enteral or parenteral nutrition and continuation of some level of physical activity is imperative in MALS patients.

Conclusion and Management

While a strong association exists between MCAS, hEDS, and POTS, coined the "trifecta," we propose that there are multiple other conditions that occur alongside this syndrome, one of which is MALS. There is no one underlying mechanism for all these conditions that has been proposed, and the link between their pathophysiology is likely multifactorial.

Patients presenting with this disease trifecta often have prior evidence of neuro-excitability and elevated sympathetic activity. Many of these patients have a history of migraines, IBS, cystitis, etc. These symptoms often developed years, if not decades, before the onset of POTS/MCAS/MALS. Thus, chronic sympathetic over-activation, perhaps starting early in life, could be part of the pathophysiology underlying these conditions. Further vagal nerve dysfunction could play a role in this sympathetic overdrive, as the vagus nerve controls heart rate, gastrointestinal motility, and other visceral functions. Additionally, it controls a neuro-inflammatory reflex, which impacts immune responses during infection or tissue injury [54]. Excessive sympathetic activity and vagal nerve dysfunction may contribute to a chronic inflammatory or autoimmune state in these patients with POTS, MCAS, MALS, GI, and autoimmune comorbidities.

Additional work on glial cells in the GI tract of animal models has revealed roles in digestion, nutrient absorption, blood flow, and immune responses. Glia are among the first cell types to respond to injury or inflammation in the gut, and tampering with enteric glial cells can create an inflammatory response [74, 75]. Glia may contribute to gut pain by secreting molecules that sensitize neurons, which is likely an adaptive response for the GI to remove anything signaling damage [76, 77]. Additionally, glia can become stressed by genetic problems, exposure to metabolites from the microbiome, poor diet, or other factors. Studies deleting the protein PIEZO2 in glial hub cells, which sense force, led to alterations in motility [76, 77]. With involvement in inflammation, hypersensitivity, and motility, glial cell modulation may be a future area of connection and investigation for patients with these chronic complex conditions.

Future Management

Overall, when approaching patients with suspected MALS, a holistic review of their symptoms and other conditions should be considered. Additionally, bringing on board the necessary specialists to manage the multiple conditions is critical. Of note, these patients may present with a long history of engagement with the medical system and extensive medical trauma. As such, these patients may be hesitant to share their concerns and experience anxiety in the evaluation. Listening to the patient's story, demonstrating compassion, and mutually defining goals of the physician-patient interaction can help set realistic expectations for the patient and help prevent physician burnout.

MCAS

We recommend all patients with concern for MCAS be seen by an allergist and worked up appropriately. From there, managing MCAS involves reducing triggers, minimizing histamine response, and trying to reduce symptom burden. We want to highlight that MCAS has defined diagnostic criteria, as described previously. However, we recognize there are challenges to appropriately diagnosing MCAS, even in symptomatic patients. For patients who do not meet all diagnostic criteria, histamine intolerance may be considered as an alternative explanation for their symptoms.

Reducing triggers in MCAS can be a complex process. Undergoing necessary immunological testing to screen for any food or environmental allergens can be helpful. Unfortunately, testing for food insensitivities is more challenging. Elimination diets are currently the gold standard for identifying any food insensitivities. It is important to work with a registered dietitian who can counsel patients on maintaining a balanced diet and keeping their caloric load high enough for their body mass during elimination diets. Once triggers have been identified, in the initial stages of disease management avoidance is ideal. Over time, based on the severity of the trigger, they can be reintroduced slowly.

In terms of minimizing histamine response and mast cell release or stimulation, pharmacological measures will likely be necessary. First-line medications include first- and second-generation antihistamines, such as loratadine, cetirizine, and fexofenadine, as well as cromolyn and vitamin C [78]. Once daily or twice daily dosing can be considered based on symptom severity. Second-line medications include immunosuppressive drugs, and the third line includes omalizumab (Xolair) [78]. Other medications that have been utilized with some success in MCAS include quercetin and cyproheptadine, among others, although there have been no therapeutic trials for medications in MCAS [78–80].

EDS

While there are no therapies currently approved to treat hEDS, early diagnosis allows for better disease monitoring and management [18]. To evaluate for EDS, a physical examination should assess joint and skin abnormalities including dislocations, subluxations, fractures, and surveillance of other issues, such as scoliosis, Chiari malformation, cervical instability, and migraines/headaches. Deconditioning may occur in these patients who have challenges with exercise and maintaining their fitness level due to lack of nutrition, pain, and symptom burden, which can further worsen laxity. Physical therapy, exercise, and lifestyle modifications are all critical steps that patients with hEDS should be encouraged to pursue. Physical therapy for hEDS is particularly crucial as exercises are targeted for managing the joint laxity and instability seen in hEDS.

As discussed previously, hEDS is associated with the presence of multiple compression syndromes. Thus, it is critical to screen for all possible abdominal compression syndromes, as correction of just one can result in worsening of symptoms. Our recommendation is to screen and treat all vascular compression syndromes (nutcracker syndrome, May–Thurner syndrome, superior mesenteric artery syndrome) in these patients.

POTS

Current therapies for POTS are primarily directed towards symptom management and control, rather than an underlying cause. Lifestyle modifications may include dietary changes, such as increasing salt and water intake, exercise programs, proper sleep hygiene, avoidance of excessive heat, and compression garments. Because patients with MALS often have limited oral intake, are on enteral or parenteral nutrition, and have additional autonomic challenges, adjustments in the approach to the treatment of POTS in MALS patients may be necessary. If nutritional intake is limited, patients should consult with their dietitian for how to optimize fluid, electrolyte, and caloric intake. Vitamin levels such as B and D vitamins should be checked and supplemented appropriately. Discussion of the risks and benefits of nutritional support including feeding tubes and IV nutrition and hydration is important early in the disease course to prevent the effects of malnutrition and dehydration.

We recommend the administration of the COMPASS 31 to screen for symptoms of panautonomic dysfunction. If patients present with symptoms of dry mouth and eyes, temperature dysregulation, Raynaud's phenomenon, sweating abnormalities, etc., they may need to be screened for other autoimmune and neurological conditions. Additionally, with the high rates of GI dysmotility seen in POTS patients, we recommend all patients undergo necessary tests and screening. Both upper and lower GI motility should be assessed via multiple modalities, such as gastric emptying studies and antroduodenal manometry for upper motility and Sitz marker studies for lower motility.

Patients with MALS may not be able to participate in typical POTS exercise programs or cardiac rehabilitation. As such, exercises should be specifically tailored to maintain as much fitness and muscle mass as possible, recognizing their limited caloric intake, with the goal of preventing exacerbations in symptoms.

Medications frequently need to be utilized in those with MALS and POTS. Medication options may include fludrocortisone (IV albumin) for increasing blood volume, midodrine or octreotide for vasoconstriction, beta-blockers or ivabradine for reducing tachycardia, SSRIs or SNRIs for improving central cardiovascular control while also helping with mood, and pyridostigmine for facilitating synapse transmission [39, 44]. Importantly, beta-blockers may need to be used with caution in patients with both POTS and MCAS, as there have been instances of increased bronchospasm severity or hypotension during anaphylactic reactions [81]. This may be because a hyperadrenergic response in POTS can lower the threshold for mast cell degranulation and cause flushing; in such cases, antihistamines should be used before trying beta blockers. Overall, the goal is that medications improve the quality of life in the interim. Eventually, treatment of underlying causes, if possible, and lifestyle modifications may allow for medication discontinuation.

References

1. Overview & Diagnosis - TMS - The Mast Cell Disease Society, Inc. https://tmsforacure.org/overview/. Accessed 10 July 2023.
2. Jackson RL. Carcinoid syndrome and disorders of systemic mast-cell activation including systemic mastocytosis. Endocrinol Metab Clin N Am. 1988;17(2):415–36. https://doi.org/10.1016/S0889-8529(18)30427-4.
3. Akin C, Valent P, Metcalfe DD. Mast cell activation syndrome: proposed diagnostic criteria. J Allergy Clin Immunol. 2010;126(6):1099–104. https://doi.org/10.1016/J.JACI.2010.08.035.
4. Leru PM, Anton VF, Ureche C, Zurac S, Bratu O, Neagoe CD. Mast cell activation syndromes - evaluation of current diagnostic criteria and laboratory tools in clinical practice. Exp Ther Med. 2020;20(3):2348. https://doi.org/10.3892/ETM.2020.8947.
5. Lyons JJ, Yu X, Hughes JD, et al. Elevated basal serum tryptase identifies a multisystem disorder associated with increased TPSAB1 copy number. Nat Genet. 2016;48(12):1564. https://doi.org/10.1038/NG.3696.
6. Hamilton MJ, Zhao M, Giannetti MP, et al. Distinct small intestine mast cell histologic changes in patients with hereditary alpha-tryptasemia and mast cell activation syndrome. Am J Surg Pathol. 2021;45(7):997. https://doi.org/10.1097/PAS.0000000000001676.
7. De Winter BY, van den Wijngaard RM, de Jonge WJ. Intestinal mast cells in gut inflammation and motility disturbances. Biochim Biophys Acta. 2012;1822(1):66–73. https://doi.org/10.1016/J.BBADIS.2011.03.016.
8. Akbar A, Yiangou Y, Facer P, Walters JRF, Anand P, Ghosh S. Increased capsaicin receptor TRPV1-expressing sensory fibres in irritable bowel syndrome and their correlation with abdominal pain. Gut. 2008;57(7):923–9. https://doi.org/10.1136/GUT.2007.138982.
9. Lee KN, Lee OY. The role of mast cells in irritable bowel syndrome. Gastroenterol Res Pract. 2016;2016:2031480. https://doi.org/10.1155/2016/2031480.
10. Bassotti G, Villanacci V, Nascimbeni R, et al. Colonic mast cells in controls and slow transit constipation patients. Aliment Pharmacol Ther. 2011;34(1):92–9. https://doi.org/10.1111/J.1365-2036.2011.04684.X.
11. Kim K. Abdominal vascular compression syndromes: current and future of management of abdominal vascular compression syndromes that includes median arcuate ligament syndrome, nutcracker syndrome, superior mesenteric artery syndrome, May–Thurner Syndrome, and associated pelvic venous insufficiency. J Vasc Surg. 2023;77(4):50S. https://doi.org/10.1016/j.jvs.2023.01.139.
12. Barbon DA, Hsu R, Noga J, Lazzara B, Miller T, Stainken BF. Clinical response to celiac plexus block confirms the neurogenic etiology of median arcuate ligament syndrome. J Vasc Interv Radiol. 2021;32(7):1081–7. https://doi.org/10.1016/J.JVIR.2021.04.003.
13. Sturiale A, Alemanno G, Giudici F, Addasi R, Bellucci F, Tonelli F. Median arcuate ligament syndrome in a patient with Crohn's disease. Int J Surg Case Rep. 2013;4(4):399–402. https://doi.org/10.1016/j.ijscr.2013.01.015.
14. Woestemeier A, Semaan A, Block A, et al. Prognostic factors for the long term outcome after surgical celiac artery decompression in MALS. Orphanet J Rare Dis. 2022;18(1):334. https://doi.org/10.21203/RS.3.RS-1844555/V1.

15. Akin C. How to evaluate the patient with a suspected mast cell disorder and how/when to manage symptoms. Hematology. 2022;2022(1):55–63. https://doi.org/10.1182/HEMATOLOGY.2022000366.
16. Valent P, Akin C, Bonadonna P, et al. Proposed diagnostic algorithm for patients with suspected mast cell activation syndrome. J Allergy Clin Immunol Pract. 2019;7(4):1125–33. https://doi.org/10.1016/J.JAIP.2019.01.006.
17. Malfait F, Francomano C, Byers P, et al. The 2017 international classification of the Ehlers–Danlos syndromes. Am J Med Genet C Semin Med Genet. 2017;175(1):8–26. https://doi.org/10.1002/AJMG.C.31552.
18. Gensemer C, Burks R, Kautz S, Judge DP, Lavallee M, Norris RA. Hypermobile Ehlers-Danlos syndromes: complex phenotypes, challenging diagnoses, and poorly understood causes. Dev Dyn. 2021;250(3):318–44. https://doi.org/10.1002/DVDY.220.
19. Demmler JC, Atkinson MD, Reinhold EJ, Choy E, Lyons RA, Brophy ST. Diagnosed prevalence of Ehlers-Danlos syndrome and hypermobility spectrum disorder in Wales, UK: a national electronic cohort study and case–control comparison. BMJ Open. 2019;9(11):e031365. https://doi.org/10.1136/BMJOPEN-2019-031365.
20. Castori M, Dordoni C, Morlino S, et al. Spectrum of mucocutaneous manifestations in 277 patients with joint hypermobility syndrome/Ehlers-Danlos syndrome, hypermobility type. Am J Med Genet C Semin Med Genet. 2015;169(1):43–53. https://doi.org/10.1002/AJMG.C.31425.
21. Castori M, Tinkle B, Levy H, Grahame R, Malfait F, Hakim A. A framework for the classification of joint hypermobility and related conditions. Am J Med Genet C Semin Med Genet. 2017;175(1):148–57. https://doi.org/10.1002/AJMG.C.31539.
22. hEDS Diagnostic Checklist - The Ehlers Danlos Society. https://www.ehlers-danlos.com/heds-diagnostic-checklist/. Accessed 10 July 2023.
23. Nelson AD, Mouchli MA, Valentin N, et al. Ehlers Danlos syndrome and gastrointestinal manifestations: a 20-year experience at Mayo Clinic. Neurogastroenterol Motil. 2015;27(11):1657–66. https://doi.org/10.1111/NMO.12665.
24. De Wandele I, Rombaut L, Malfait F, De Backer T, De Paepe A, Calders P. Clinical heterogeneity in patients with the hypermobility type of Ehlers-Danlos syndrome. Res Dev Disabil. 2013;34(3):873–81. https://doi.org/10.1016/J.RIDD.2012.11.018.
25. Zeitoun JD, Lefèvre JH, De Parades V, et al. Functional digestive symptoms and quality of life in patients with Ehlers-Danlos syndromes: results of a National Cohort Study on 134 patients. PLoS One. 2013;8(11):e80321. https://doi.org/10.1371/JOURNAL.PONE.0080321.
26. Huynh DTK, Shamash K, Burch M, et al. Median arcuate ligament syndrome and its associated conditions. Am Surg. 2019;85(10):1162–5. https://doi.org/10.1177/000313481908501019.
27. Diagnosis and treatment of vascular compression syndromes of the abdomen based on the anatomical features of man and gender-specific characteristics after puberty content.
28. Shirley ED, DeMaio M, Bodurtha J. Ehlers-Danlos syndrome in orthopaedics: etiology, diagnosis, and treatment implications. Sports Health. 2012;4(5):394. https://doi.org/10.1177/1941738112452385.
29. Hansen AJ, Toker A, Hayanga J, Buenaventura P, Spear C, Abbas G. Minimally invasive repair of adult slipped rib syndrome without costal cartilage excision. Ann Thorac Surg. 2020;110(3):1030–5. https://doi.org/10.1016/j.athoracsur.2020.02.081.
30. Khan NA, Waseem S, Ullah S, Mehmood H. Slipping rib syndrome in a female adult with longstanding intractable upper abdominal pain. Case Rep Med. 2018;2018:7484560. https://doi.org/10.1155/2018/7484560.
31. Robb L, Robb M. The slipping rib syndrome: an overlooked cause of abdominal pain. Pract Pain Manage. 2014;13:7.
32. Wells R, Spurrier AJ, Linz D, et al. Postural tachycardia syndrome: current perspectives. Vasc Health Risk Manag. 2018;14:1. https://doi.org/10.2147/VHRM.S127393.
33. Agarwal AK, Garg R, Ritch A, Sarkar P. Postural orthostatic tachycardia syndrome. Postgrad Med J. 2007;83(981):478. https://doi.org/10.1136/PGMJ.2006.055046.

34. Sheldon RS, Grubb BP, Olshansky B, et al. 2015 Heart Rhythm Society Expert consensus statement on the diagnosis and treatment of postural tachycardia syndrome, inappropriate sinus tachycardia, and vasovagal syncope. Heart Rhythm. 2015;12(6):e41–63. https://doi.org/10.1016/J.HRTHM.2015.03.029.
35. Vernino S, Bourne KM, Stiles LE, et al. Postural orthostatic tachycardia syndrome (POTS): state of the science and clinical care from a 2019 National Institutes of Health Expert Consensus Meeting - part 1. Auton Neurosci. 2021;235:102828. https://doi.org/10.1016/J.AUTNEU.2021.102828.
36. Arnold AC, Ng J, Raj SR. Postural tachycardia syndrome – diagnosis, physiology, and prognosis. Auton Neurosci. 2018;215:3–11. https://doi.org/10.1016/J.AUTNEU.2018.02.005.
37. Mathias CJ, Low DA, Iodice V, et al. Postural tachycardia syndrome—current experience and concepts. Nat Rev Neurol. 2011;8(1):22–34. https://doi.org/10.1038/nrneurol.2011.187.
38. Zhang R, Mayuga K, Shields R, Cantrell C, Wilson R. Skin biopsy and quantitative sudomotor axon reflex testing in patients with postural orthostatic tachycardia syndrome. Cureus. 2022;14(11):31021. https://doi.org/10.7759/CUREUS.31021.
39. Kavi L, Gammage MD, Grubb BP, Karabin BL. Postural tachycardia syndrome: multiple symptoms, but easily missed. Br J Gen Pract. 2012;62(599):286. https://doi.org/10.3399/BJGP12X648963.
40. Raj SR. The postural tachycardia syndrome (POTS): pathophysiology, diagnosis & management. Indian Pacing Electrophysiol J. 2006;6(2):84.
41. Gwathmey KG. Sensory polyneuropathies. Continuum Lifelong Learn Neurol. 2017;23(5):1411–36. https://doi.org/10.1212/CON.0000000000000518.
42. Igharo D, Thiel JC, Rolke R, et al. Skin biopsy reveals generalized small fibre neuropathy in hypermobile Ehlers–Danlos syndromes. Eur J Neurol. 2023;30(3):719–28. https://doi.org/10.1111/ENE.15649.
43. Ruzieh M, Grubb BP. Orthostatic intolerance and postural tachycardia syndrome: new insights into pathophysiology and treatment. Herzschrittmacherther Elektrophysiol. 2018;29(2):183–6. https://doi.org/10.1007/S00399-018-0563-1/METRICS.
44. Tooba R, Mayuga KA, Wilson R, Tonelli AR. Dyspnea in chronic low ventricular preload states. Ann Am Thorac Soc. 2021;18(4):573–81.
45. Kohno R, Cannom DS, Olshansky B, et al. Mast cell activation disorder and postural orthostatic tachycardia syndrome: a clinical association. J Am Heart Assoc. 2021;10(17):21002. https://doi.org/10.1161/JAHA.121.021002.
46. Garland EM, Celedonio JE, Raj SR. Postural tachycardia syndrome: beyond orthostatic intolerance. Curr Neurol Neurosci Rep. 2015;15(9):60. https://doi.org/10.1007/S11910-015-0583-8.
47. Shibao C, Arzubiaga C, Roberts LJ, et al. Hyperadrenergic postural tachycardia syndrome in mast cell activation disorders. Hypertension. 2005;45(3):385–90. https://doi.org/10.1161/01.HYP.0000158259.68614.40.
48. Shaw BH, Stiles LE, Bourne K, et al. The face of postural tachycardia syndrome – insights from a large cross-sectional online community-based survey. J Intern Med. 2019;286(4):438–48. https://doi.org/10.1111/JOIM.12895.
49. Fedorowski A. Postural orthostatic tachycardia syndrome: clinical presentation, aetiology and management. J Intern Med. 2019;285(4):352–66. https://doi.org/10.1111/JOIM.12852.
50. Li X, Raventós B, Roel E, et al. Association between covid-19 vaccination, SARS-CoV-2 infection, and risk of immune mediated neurological events: population based cohort and self-controlled case series analysis. BMJ. 2022;376:e068373. https://doi.org/10.1136/BMJ-2021-068373.
51. Parker WH, Moudgil R, Wilson RG, Tonelli AR, Mayuga KA, Singh TK. COVID-19 and postural tachycardia syndrome: a case series. Eur Heart J Case Rep. 2021;5(12):ytab325. https://doi.org/10.1093/EHJCR/YTAB325.
52. Goldstein DS. The possible association between COVID-19 and postural tachycardia syndrome. Heart Rhythm. 2021;18(4):508. https://doi.org/10.1016/J.HRTHM.2020.12.007.

53. Weinstock LB, Brook JB, Myers TL, Goodman B. Successful treatment of postural orthostatic tachycardia and mast cell activation syndromes using naltrexone, immunoglobulin and antibiotic treatment. Case Rep Dermatol. 2018;2018:221405. https://doi.org/10.1136/BCR-2017-221405.
54. Vernino S, Stiles LE. Autoimmunity in postural orthostatic tachycardia syndrome: current understanding. Auton Neurosci. 2018;215:78–82. https://doi.org/10.1016/J.AUTNEU.2018.04.005.
55. Penny HA, Aziz I, Ferrar M, et al. Is there a relationship between gluten sensitivity and postural tachycardia syndrome? Eur J Gastroenterol Hepatol. 2016;28(12):1383–7. https://doi.org/10.1097/MEG.0000000000000740.
56. Pasadyn SR, Warren CB, Wilson RG. Utility of salivary gland biopsy in diagnosing Sjogren's syndrome in a POTS patient population. Auton Neurosci. 2020;227:102694. https://doi.org/10.1016/j.autneu.2020.102694.
57. Watari M, Nakane S, Mukaino A, et al. Autoimmune postural orthostatic tachycardia syndrome. Ann Clin Transl Neurol. 2018;5(4):486–92. https://doi.org/10.1002/ACN3.524.
58. Rea NA, Campbell CL, Cortez MM. Quantitative assessment of autonomic symptom burden in postural tachycardia syndrome (POTS). J Neurol Sci. 2017;377:35–41. https://doi.org/10.1016/J.JNS.2017.03.032.
59. Wang LB, Culbertson CJ, Deb A, Morgenshtern K, Huang H, Hohler AD. Gastrointestinal dysfunction in postural tachycardia syndrome. J Neurol Sci. 2015;359(1-2):193–6. https://doi.org/10.1016/J.JNS.2015.10.052.
60. Zhang LN, Moak JP, Desbiens J, et al. Utility of diagnostic studies for upper gastrointestinal symptoms in children with orthostatic intolerance. J Pediatr. 2019;205:138–44. https://doi.org/10.1016/j.jpeds.2018.09.048.
61. Loavenbruck A, Iturrino J, Singer W, et al. Disturbances of gastrointestinal transit and autonomic functions in postural orthostatic tachycardia syndrome. Neurogastroenterol Motil. 2015;27(1):92–8. https://doi.org/10.1111/NMO.12480.
62. DiBaise JK, Harris LA, Goodman B. Postural tachycardia syndrome (POTS) and the GI tract: a primer for the Gastroenterologist. Am J Gastroenterol. 2018;113(10):1458–67. https://doi.org/10.1038/S41395-018-0215-4.
63. Candal R, Reddy V, Samra NS. Anatomy, abdomen and pelvis, celiac ganglia. Treasure Island: StatPearls Publishing; 2020.
64. DeCicco J, Raja F, Ganesan S, El-Hayek K. First description of a histopathologic grading system and relationship to outcomes after robotic median arcuate ligament release with celiac ganglionectomy and lymphadenectomy. Surgery. 2024;175(3):822–32. https://doi.org/10.1016/J.SURG.2023.09.024.
65. Weber JM, Boules M, Fong K, et al. Median arcuate ligament syndrome is not a vascular disease. Ann Vasc Surg. 2016;30:22–7. https://doi.org/10.1016/j.avsg.2015.07.013.
66. Bech FR. Celiac artery compression syndromes. Surg Clin N Am. 1997;77(2):409–24. https://doi.org/10.1016/S0039-6109(05)70558-2.
67. Coss-Adame E, Rao SSC. Brain and gut interactions in irritable Bowel syndrome: new paradigms and new understandings. Curr Gastroenterol Rep. 2014;16(4):379. https://doi.org/10.1007/S11894-014-0379-Z.
68. Midenfjord I, Polster A, Sjövall H, Friberg P, Törnblom H, Simrén M. Associations among neurophysiology measures in irritable bowel syndrome (IBS) and their relevance for IBS symptoms. Sci Rep. 2020;10(1):1–11. https://doi.org/10.1038/s41598-020-66558-w.
69. Ashangari C, Suleman A, Le TH. Median arcuate ligament syndrome in postural orthostatic tachycardia syndrome (POTS). Auton Neurosci. 2015;192:124–5. https://doi.org/10.1016/J.AUTNEU.2015.07.225.
70. Kalapatapu V. Median arcuate ligament syndrome and concomitant autonomic dysfunction pathology—case reports and Penn treatment algorithm. J Vasc Surg. 2022;75(6):e195–6. https://doi.org/10.1016/j.jvs.2022.03.379.

71. Moak JP, Ramwell C, Fabian R, Hanumanthaiah S, Darbari A, Kane TD. Median arcuate ligament syndrome with orthostatic intolerance: intermediate-term outcomes following surgical intervention. J Pediatr. 2021;231:141–7. https://doi.org/10.1016/J.JPEDS.2020.12.024.
72. Abdallah H, Thammineni K, Hartas G, Kane K. Median arcuate ligament syndrome presenting as POTS. Auton Neurosci. 2015;192:123. https://doi.org/10.1016/j.autneu.2015.07.220.
73. Fu Q, VanGundy TB, Galbreath MM, et al. Cardiac origins of the postural orthostatic tachycardia syndrome. J Am Coll Cardiol. 2010;55(25):2858–68. https://doi.org/10.1016/J.JACC.2010.02.043.
74. Morales-Soto W, Gonzales J, Jackson WF, Gulbransen BD. Enteric glia promote visceral hypersensitivity during inflammation through intercellular signaling with gut nociceptors. Sci Signal. 2023;16:812. https://doi.org/10.1126/SCISIGNAL.ADG1668.
75. Le Berre C, Naveilhan P, Rolli-Derkinderen M. Enteric glia at center stage of inflammatory bowel disease. Neurosci Lett. 2023;809:137315. https://doi.org/10.1016/j.neulet.2023.137315.
76. Scavuzzo MA, Letai KC, Maeno-Hikichi Y, et al. Enteric glial hub cells coordinate intestinal motility. bioRxiv. 2023. https://doi.org/10.1101/2023.06.07.544052.
77. Scavuzzo M. The way you move. Science. 2023;382(6670):527–8.
78. Molderings GJ, Haenisch B, Brettner S, et al. Pharmacological treatment options for mast cell activation disease. Naunyn Schmiedeberg's Arch Pharmacol. 2016;389(7):671–94. https://doi.org/10.1007/S00210-016-1247-1.
79. Weng Z, Zhang B, Asadi S, et al. Quercetin is more effective than cromolyn in blocking human mast cell cytokine release and inhibits contact dermatitis and photosensitivity in humans. PLoS One. 2012;7(3):33805. https://doi.org/10.1371/JOURNAL.PONE.0033805.
80. Maintz L, Novak N. Histamine and histamine intolerance. Am J Clin Nutr. 2007;85(5):1185–96. https://doi.org/10.1093/AJCN/85.5.1185.
81. Bonamichi-Santos R, Yoshimi-Kanamori K, Giavina-Bianchi P, Aun MV. Association of postural tachycardia syndrome and Ehlers-Danlos syndrome with mast cell activation disorders. Immunol Allergy Clin N Am. 2018;38(3):497–504. https://doi.org/10.1016/J.IAC.2018.04.004.

Chapter 7
Vascular Compressions and Syndromes Associated with Median Arcuate Ligament Syndrome: May-Thurner, Nutcracker, and Pelvic Congestion Syndrome

Natalie Chao, Eleanor Dunlap, Joshua Plant, and Khanjan H. Nagarsheth

Introduction

Vascular compression syndromes of the abdomen and pelvis are anatomic variations that can cause extrinsic compression of specific veins and the gastrointestinal tract. These compressions can manifest alongside median arcuate ligament syndrome (MALS) and can similarly cause chronic pain, malnutrition, and a variety of other symptoms, as well as the development of venous thromboses. These conditions present nonspecifically and are exceedingly uncommon, which creates a major challenge in diagnosis; however, the timely recognition of these syndromes is essential, and an appropriate diagnostic algorithm must be followed to delineate a comprehensive treatment plan for the patient.

Herein, the authors will describe the most common vascular compression syndromes routinely found in the abdomen and pelvis. This chapter will delineate left renal vein compression or nutcracker syndrome (NCS), left common iliac vein compression or May-Thurner syndrome (MTS), and pelvic congestion syndrome (PCS). A comprehensive review of these compressions associated with MALS, including the etiology, clinical presentation, diagnostic algorithm, and various treatment options, will be presented below.

N. Chao
School of Medicine, University of Maryland, Baltimore, MD, USA

E. Dunlap · J. Plant
Division of Vascular Surgery, University of Maryland Medical Center, Baltimore, MD, USA

K. H. Nagarsheth (✉)
School of Medicine, University of Maryland, Baltimore, MD, USA

Division of Vascular Surgery, University of Maryland Medical Center, Baltimore, MD, USA
e-mail: KNagarsheth@som.umaryland.edu

D. Shouhed et al. (eds.), *Median Arcuate Ligament Syndrome*,
https://doi.org/10.1007/978-3-031-80740-4_7

Nutcracker Syndrome (Left Renal Vein Entrapment Syndrome)

Etiology

Left renal vein (LRV) entrapment syndrome or nutcracker syndrome (NCS) is caused by compression of the left renal vein by surrounding structures, leading to stenosis of the aortomesenteric region of the LRV and dilatation of the distal portion of the LRV [1]. LRV was first referred to as nutcracker syndrome by de Schepper, who compared the compression of the vein to that of a nutcracker shutting [2]. It is most commonly the result of entrapment between the SMA and aorta, where it is coined anterior nutcracker [3]. Anterior NCS can manifest in patients with low body weight from the reduction of adipose tissue narrowing the aortomesenteric angle. It can also be seen in patients with lordosis or scoliosis, renal ptosis, vascular abnormalities, and intraabdominal tumors [4].

A less common variant that compresses the retro-aortic or circum-aortic artery between the aorta and the vertebral body is termed posterior nutcracker [5, 6]. Posterior NCS is most commonly caused by pathologies, such as aneurysms or osteophytosis, and can occasionally occur as a result of aortomesenteric angle narrowing secondary to Wilkie syndrome [7]. Ehlers-Danlos syndrome and mast cell activation syndrome have also been associated with increased rates of NCS [8]. Young adults, particularly young women, are most affected.

Inherited NCS is caused by irregularities in embryological LRV development from the aortic collar at 6–8 weeks gestation [9]. Anterior anastomosis of the aortic collar with anterior, supra, and subcardinal veins develop the LRV while the posterior anastomosis normally degenerates. Degeneration of the anterior anastomosis instead of the posterior can lead to retro-aortic LRV, and failure to degenerate the posterior can create circum-aortic LRV. The normal aortomesenteric angle is greater than 22°, and the normal distance between the two vessels is less than 8 mm. There is no standard distance between the aorta and spine that serves as a cutoff for posterior NCS diagnosis. The term NCS specifically refers to the symptomatic presentation of LRV entrapment. LRV compression with associated hemodynamics that does not present with clinical symptoms is characterized as nutcracker phenomenon [3, 10].

Clinical Presentation

Symptoms of NCS are variable and nonspecific, which increases the difficulty of diagnosis. Hematuria, left flank pain, and abdominal pain are the most classic triad of symptoms and are defined as the typical subtype [11]. Hematuria is often the first symptom and is caused by the rupture of thin varices due to increased venous pressure from compression of the pelvic collecting vessels. Microhematuria is up to four times more common than macrohematuria [3, 10]. Proteinuria can also be detected on urinalysis [3]. Pain is the second most common symptom. Abdominal, left back, and left flank pain from venous hypertension can radiate to the thigh and buttocks and may be exacerbated by certain positioning [12]. Left flank pain can be further worsened by left ureteral colic as a result of venous thrombus from renal congestion passing down the ureter [3].

The atypical subtype of NCS includes urologic features. Left RV varices and gonadal varices caused by LRV compression lead to pelvic congestion syndrome (PCS), which is characterized by ovarian vein reflux or outflow obstruction leading to localized pain. Dyspareunia and dysmenorrhea can also manifest secondary to congestion. Physical examination may show vulvar and pelvic varices and tortuous lower extremity varicosities. Varicoceles in male patients follow a similar pathophysiology. Reflux or obstruction of the testicular vein from LRV compression causes dilation of the pampiniform plexus and resultant pain. However, varicocele is less common than PCS [13].

Early satiety, nausea, weight loss, and postprandial pain have also been associated with NCS, but gastric symptoms are usually reported in patients with concurrent SMA syndrome or Wilkie syndrome [14]. Systemic symptoms such as headache, hypotension, syncope, and tachycardia may also occur, albeit rarely, and may be a sign of associated conditions, such as postural orthostatic tachycardia syndrome (POTS) [4, 15].

Diagnosis

The diagnosis of NCS requires taking into consideration a comprehensive medical history with an emphasis on symptom presentation and risk factors, as well as an accurate interpretation of laboratory studies and imaging findings, to create a full clinical picture (Fig. 7.1). A detailed history should be collected to assess the timing of symptom onset, severity, and any precipitating factors such as associated comorbidities. Presentation of hematuria with chronic abdominal and flank pain should immediately heighten suspicion, especially in underweight young patients [16]. Physical examination should include inspection for pelvic varices and thin body habitus. In the setting of sudden onset hematuria, more common renal conditions should be ruled out via urinalysis, urine culture, cytology, urethrocystoscopy, CT urography, renal ultrasound, and finally renal biopsy [3].

Diagnosis of NCS is often by exclusion and is confirmed with an array of imaging studies, including Doppler ultrasound, venography, and intravascular ultrasound (IVUS) [7]. Doppler ultrasound is the most prevalent first-line imaging method employed in clinical practice because it shows the aortomesenteric angle and

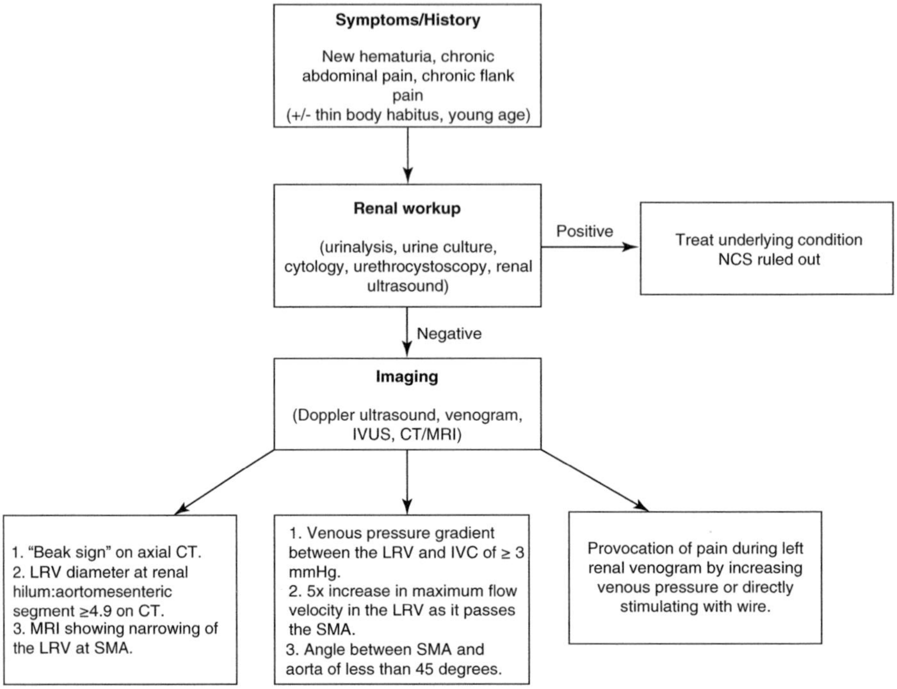

Fig. 7.1 Diagnostic algorithm flow diagram of NCS

distance, congestion of LRV flow, and degree of LRV stenosis [7]. While this is beneficial for anterior NCS, it does not show duodenal compression, and so CT should be integrated for patients suspicious of posterior NCS. Catheter venography with renal vein IVUS is the gold standard for establishing diagnosis, but its invasiveness makes it less desirable for young patients [13].

Proposed diagnostic criteria include the following: (1) venous pressure gradient between the LRV and IVC of $\geq$3 mmHg; (2) fivefold increase in maximum flow velocity in the LRV as it passes the SMA; (3) angle between SMA and aorta of less than 45° [17]; however, the data supporting these criteria is sparse and inconsistent. A ratio of LRV diameter at the renal hilum to diameter at the aortomesenteric segment $\geq$4.9 on CT has also been reported to have high specificity for NCS [18]. Magnetic resonance imaging (MRI) is preferred for children and adolescents due to the lack of radiation exposure and the ability to examine adjacent structures, such as the gonadal veins [18, 19]. A "beak sign" in the axial plane of CT and MRI showing abrupt narrowing of the LRV at the SMA is a highly sensitive and specific sign of anterior NCS [19].

The authors of this chapter add provocation of pain during LRV venogram as a diagnostic criterion for left renal vein entrapment syndrome. Stimulating pain in the renal hilar nerves by increasing pressure within the left renal vein or by direct stimulation with a stiff wire has shown significant prognostic benefit. If identical symptoms are not reproduced during a provocative venogram, improvement following surgery for NCS is less likely, and other sources of symptoms must be considered.

Treatment

There is a lack of standardized guidelines for the management of NCS due to limited data. Treatment is therefore individually determined by scaling the severity of symptoms and can range in invasiveness from close monitoring to full nephrectomy. Treatment via conservative medical management is recommended for mild symptoms. Surgical treatment is reserved for patients with severe symptoms or if symptoms persist for more than 6 months in adults and greater than 24 months in children [20]. The main objectives of surgical treatment are to reduce venous hypertension and secondarily reduce any pelvic venous reflux.

Conservative medical treatment should be considered for patients under 18 years of age with only discrete hematuria and mild symptoms [21]. Younger patients may still be growing, and so completion of the LRV, SMA, aorta, and surrounding collateral development may self-resolve compression. Adults should receive conservative treatment under closer observation for at least 6 months prior to considering any interventions. Low-dose aspirin can help with renal perfusion and angiotensin-converting enzyme inhibitors, particularly alacepril, can alleviate orthostatic proteinuria [22]. Encouraging weight gain is recommended to increase the aortomesenteric angle, and compression stockings can relieve some of the congestion causing pelvic and flank pain [23].

LRV transposition is the most common and preferred surgical treatment for both anterior and posterior NCS. It involves transposition of the LRV distally to the inferior vena cava (IVC) via a midline transperitoneal approach [24]. The small and large intestines are moved aside, and the duodenum is mobilized to the ligament of Treitz so that the retroperitoneum can enter midline and inferior to the transverse mesocolon [20]. The aorta, LRV, and IVC are then identified, and the connective tissue between the SMA and aorta is dissected so that the LRV can be mobilized. The IVC is also isolated at its confluence with the LRV so that the LRV can be transected with an IVC rim. The LRV is then attached as distally as possible to the left lateral aspect of the IVC. The great saphenous vein (GSV) can be used as an extension graft or patch for patients with LRV experiencing distortion or excessive tension [20]. There is a shorter period of renal ischemia and fewer anastomoses with this technique compared to other methods. Postoperative risk is low, and complications, while uncommon, include deep venous thrombosis, retroperitoneal hematoma, ileus, and intestinal obstruction by adhesions. This method has been reported to be particularly effective in resolving hematuria and flank pain and has been lauded as the gold standard treatment for NCS [1, 25, 26].

Left renal autotransplantation is the second most common treatment method. It is a highly invasive but effective procedure characterized by nephrectomy and replacement of the kidney into the ipsilateral or contralateral iliac fossa. This method alleviates the discomfort caused by both LRV hypertension and any renal ptosis, leading to significantly reduced or resolved pain. While there is overall low morbidity, there are increased risks due to the longer period of renal ischemia, anastomoses of the ureter and renal artery, and more extensive dissection [20].

Simple nephropexy is no longer recommended as a sole treatment method because it only targets renal ptosis discomfort and not the symptoms directly induced by LRV compression. Nephropexy performed through a retroperitoneal approach alongside LRV transposition is an accepted compound procedure that is recommended for younger patients because of the low risk of injury to intraperitoneal organs [27].

Superior mesenteric artery transposition divides the SMA and reimplants it onto the aorta below the LRV. This transposition requires less retroperitoneal exposure and reduces the chance of thrombosis in the LRV, but it is more complex than LRV transposition and carries a higher risk for arterial thrombosis and mesenteric ischemia. Therefore, it is rarely performed [20].

Two methods of vascular bypass have been implemented, but as relatively novel or uncommon procedures, there is little available data on long-term outcomes or procedure experience [20, 21, 24]. Renocaval bypass uses autologous GSV to create a bypass. The GSV graft loops under the LRV and is attached via two anastomoses, one proximally onto the IVC and the other distally onto the LRV [28]. As a relatively novel procedure, gonadocaval bypass involves ligation of the gonadal vein and gonadal vein transposition or bypass to the IVC, which relieves pelvic congestion in addition to LRV hypertension.

Open surgery is higher risk due to its invasive nature and increased odds of infection, yet it is also regarded as a curative treatment [21]. As a result, several endovascular treatments have been introduced. Stenting has been rapidly increasing in popularity as a minimally invasive alternative to surgical treatment. It is often preferred as the primary treatment option in centers with the ability to perform an endovascular approach because of the lower risk of complications and decreased length of renal ischemia. Stenting is also performed as a secondary treatment for patients who still experience stenosis after LRV transposition [20]. Ultimately the decision to proceed with open versus endovascular surgical procedure is a multifactorial decision, depending on the patient's anatomy, comorbid conditions, and surgeon preference.

Percutaneous access is obtained via either of the common femoral veins or the right internal jugular vein. Intravascular ultrasound (IVUS) and/or venography can be employed to establish diagnosis as well as to measure the renal vein for appropriate stent sizing. Self-expanding stents (Wallstent™; Boston Scientific Corporation) 14–16 mm in diameter and 6–8 cm in length are most common and are advised to be 20% larger than the venous diameter at the renal hilum to prevent migration [21, 27]. The wire is threaded into the left gonadal vein so that the sheath can be positioned across the stenosis. The wire is then retracted into the renal vein where the stent is centered across the stenosis and finally deployed. Balloon catheter angioplasty may be necessary for full expansion of the stent if stenosis persists; however, it is usually not necessary and ideally avoided [29]. Patients should take anticoagulant and antiplatelet medications for 2–3 months after the procedure. The standard regimen is dual antiplatelet therapy for 90 days on clopidogrel and aspirin followed by lifelong aspirin. Complications include inappropriate stent placement, displacement of stent into the IVC or renal hilum region, or device migration, with embolization or thrombosis being exceedingly uncommon [21]. These complications are usually due to incorrect placement or sizing of the stent or errors in technical ability [20] (Fig. 7.2).

Gonadal vein embolization is another endovascular technique used for NCS patients with predominantly pelvic congestion symptoms. Percutaneous femoral access is more commonly used than jugular access, and appropriate imaging should be performed to monitor for renal congestion [30]. This technique may serve as an adjunct procedure for patients undergoing LRV transposition or LRV stenting.

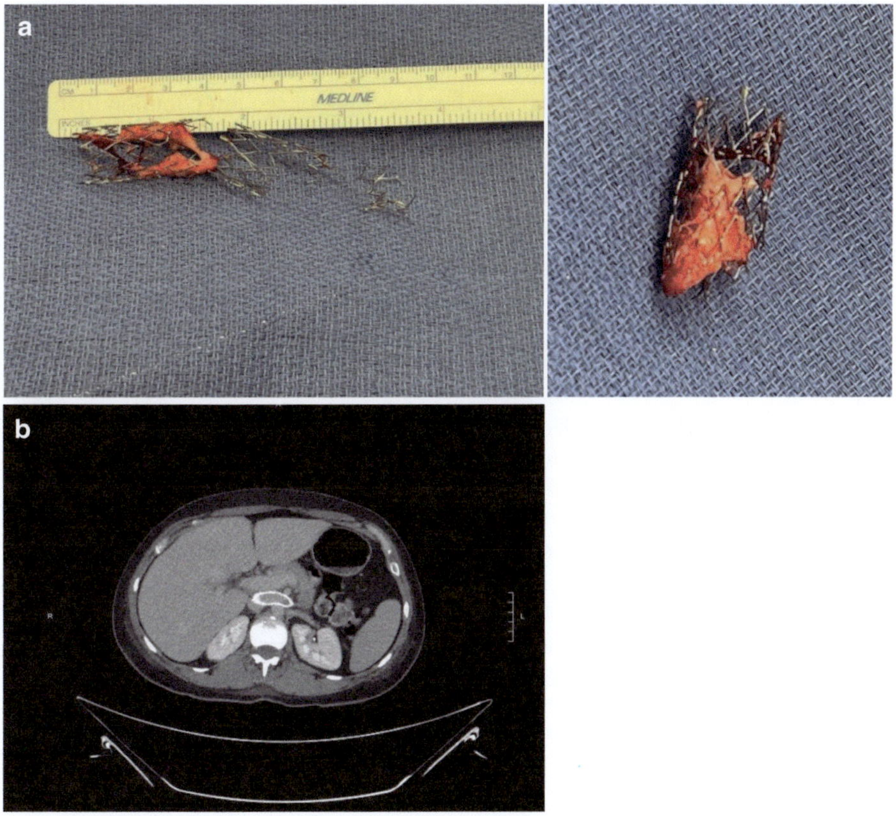

Fig. 7.2 (**a**) Explanted stent and (**b**) intravascular stent visualized on CT placed via endovascular treatment, which migrated across the inferior vena cava (Photos courtesy of Dr. KH Nagarsheth MD)

May-Thurner Syndrome (MTS)

History

May-Thurner syndrome (MTS) or left iliac vein (LIV) compression syndrome refers to compression of the left common iliac vein by the right common iliac artery against the vertebral body. Virchow was the first to report on an increased incidence of left iliofemoral thrombosis in cadavers, where the right common iliac artery compressed the left iliofemoral vein [31]. The anatomic variation of LIV compression was first fully described by two researchers, May and Thurner in 1957, who found 22% of cadavers they were studying exhibited an anatomical variant with localized intraluminal fibrous bands, referred to as spurs, on the left common iliac vein [32].

Etiology

MTS is caused by compression of the left common iliac vein by the right common iliac artery as it bifurcates from the abdominal aorta. The most common location of this extrinsic compression is at the proximal opening of the left common iliac vein just where the right common iliac artery crosses over [33]. This leads to the narrowing of the anterior-posterior diameter of the LIV as the transverse diameter widens [34]. Due to the outflow obstruction, pressure develops in the vein as it is compressed between the artery and vertebral body, leading to the formation of venous spurs [32, 35]. The compression is thought to aggravate the endothelium within the vein leading to cell proliferation and the development of spurs within the left common iliac vein.

While most cases of MTS result from congenital anatomic variations, there are also cases of acquired MTS. Spine osteophytes, aneurysmal changes, and pelvic masses, such as uterine fibroids, can lead to acquired MTS [36]. Other risk factors such as immobilization, dehydration, surgery, or hormonal changes in the setting of LIV compression can increase the risk of thrombus development [37, 38]. Females are more commonly predisposed to LIV compression due to the shape of the female pelvis. This essentially creates a prominent lumbar curvature that pushes the lower lumbar vertebrae anteriorly toward the pelvis, which can compress the LIV against the right common iliac artery [39]. Patients may remain asymptomatic due to the development of collateral veins within the pelvis that offload the narrowed left common iliac vein. This can result in the diagnosis being delayed or missed until symptoms manifest.

Clinical Presentation

The diagnosis of MTS is often delayed until venous congestion leads to the development of chronic changes around the peripheral tissues or venous thrombosis within the vein. There is a lengthy asymptomatic period of LIV compression followed by the gradual development of venous spurs or intraluminal fibrous bands. This can subsequently produce an acute unilateral left iliofemoral DVT, which can then lead to the development of a pulmonary embolism [40, 41].

Symptoms typically include left lower extremity edema, leg heaviness, and pain, which occurs regardless of gender. Over time, venous ulcerations and varicose veins can develop as a result of chronic venous hypertension [35]. The exact prevalence of MTS is unknown since some patients may be asymptomatic, but Heller et al. noted that 31% of patients with iliofemoral DVT carried a diagnosis of MTS [42]. One meta-analysis found that 46% of patients who underwent thrombolysis for clot burden within the iliofemoral system revealed an underlying iliac vein compression [43].

While traditional MTS presents with left lower extremity symptoms, there are rare cases of right-sided symptoms as a result of specific variations in vessel anatomy or enlargement of pelvic structures leading to compression [44]. Dunlap et al. reported three patients whose right lower extremity symptoms were relieved after treatment of the LIV compression [45].

Diagnosis

The diagnosis of MTS is based on clinical exam and diagnostic testing. Vascular duplex ultrasound, computed tomography (CT), and magnetic resonance imaging (MRI) allow for the evaluation of the central venous system [37]. Duplex ultrasound is safe and effective at identifying iliac vein compression, but findings can be variable based on the technical expertise of the sonographer [46, 47]. Even a skilled sonographer may be unable to visualize the iliac veins in roughly 20% of cases [48]. A negative duplex ultrasound does not conclusively rule out MTS in a symptomatic patient.

Iliac vein compression can be identified on a CT scan, along with the advantage of identifying other structural abnormalities in the lower abdomen or pelvis [49]. CT can also be helpful in ruling out other causes of left lower extremity edema including venous obstruction from underlying malignancy, hematoma, and cellulitis [41]. The static nature of CT does not allow for control over the volume status of the patient, which can lead to overdiagnosis of MTS due to dehydration [37, 41]. While CT has a high sensitivity and specificity in confirming MTS diagnosis [50], MRI can be used instead of CT in patients with renal insufficiency or an allergy to contrast media [51].

Venography with intravascular ultrasound (IVUS) is the gold standard for diagnosing MTS [37, 52] (Fig. 7.3). The real-time information obtained about the LIV diameter, integrity of the luminal wall, thrombus, and degree of compression can all be obtained without the use of contrast media by using IVUS [53]. For patients undergoing thrombectomy or stenting, the use of venography with IVUS is ideal due to its benefits of concurrent treatment of MTS [54]. The data that IVUS provides allows for accurate stent sizing, which minimizes the chance of stent migration. Before stent deployment, IVUS allows for visualization of the iliac vein confluence, assisting in accurate stent deployment and reducing the chance that the stent may obstruct the right CIV [53].

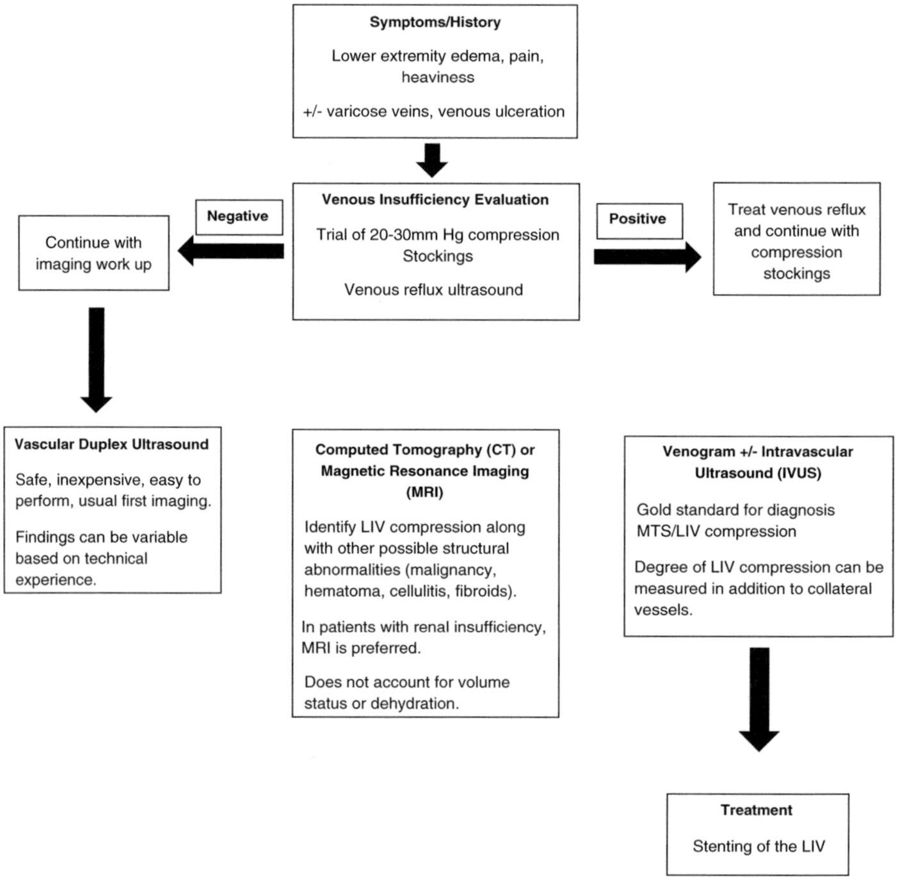

Fig. 7.3 Diagnostic algorithm flow diagram MTS

Treatment

Asymptomatic patients or those with mild symptoms of MTS may not seek medical treatment and simply manage symptoms of swelling. For symptomatic patients, minimally invasive treatment, such as angioplasty or stenting of the venous compression, relieves the outflow obstruction and provides symptom relief with good long-term patency rates [41, 55, 56] (Fig. 7.4). A 70% iliofemoral compression on IVUS has been reported to signify severe stenosis in patients with a left iliofemoral DVT [57]; however, DVTs have been reported in patients with less than 70% iliofemoral compression as well [58]. Mousa et al. noted that symptomatic MTS patients with extensive thrombosis who underwent thrombolysis followed by endovascular stenting were successfully treated 91% of the time [47]. Venography with

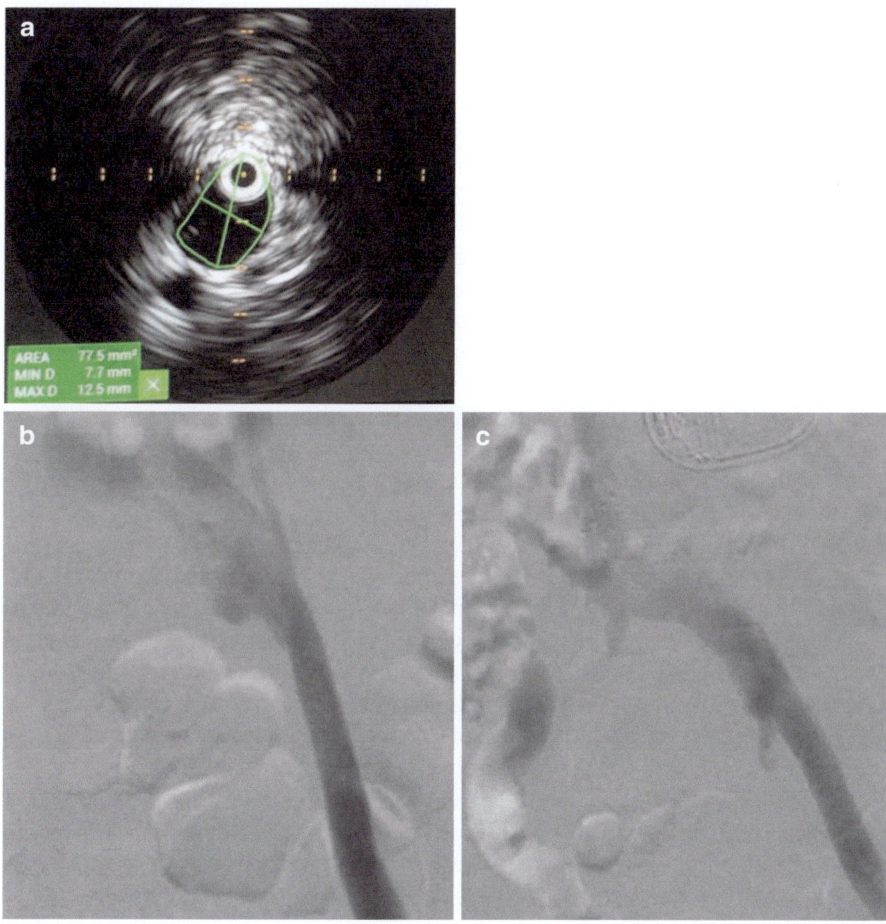

Fig. 7.4 (**a**) Venogram with IVUS. (**b**) Venogram before and after left common iliac vein stenting (Photos courtesy of Dr. KH Nagarsheth MD)

IVUS assists in accurate stent deployment, reducing the chance the stent may obstruct the right CIV leading to right lower extremity symptoms [53]. In patients with DVT from MTS, reduction of thrombus load and resolving the outflow obstruction is the cornerstone of surgical management [59]. For those with venous thrombosis, rates of post-thrombotic syndrome are reduced with endovascular treatment of the LIV compression [55].

Pelvic Congestion Syndrome (PCS)

Etiology

Chronic pelvic pain in females of reproductive age can be caused by pelvic congestion syndrome or PCS, a condition affecting millions of women worldwide. The underlying cause of PCS is pelvic venous insufficiency from retrograde venous flow in the gonadal or internal iliac veins [60, 61]. Pelvic varicose veins were first reported by the French surgeon Richet in 1957, who was the first to associate chronic pelvic pain with the presence of varicose veins in the utero-ovarian plexus [62]. Chidekel was able to use venography to demonstrate retrograde filling of the left ovarian vein as a possible cause for the development of pelvic varicosities [63].

PCS is caused by pelvic venous insufficiency leading to pelvic venous hypertension and varicosities from incompetent veins in the pelvis [60]. The venous network in the pelvis has a multitude of interconnections including connections to the hemorrhoidal, ovarian, and sacral venous plexuses. There are also connections between the pelvic veins and the superficial veins in the lower extremities. Venous hypertension caused by incompetent drainage of these veins can result in venous reflux and varicosity formation in the pelvis leading to symptoms of pain and pressure [64].

While the exact etiology of PCS is unknown, it is believed that venous congestion is due to a combination of hormones, insufficiency of the venous system, and venous obstruction [65]. During pregnancy, veins can expand up to 50% the normal size to support the developing fetus. These changes to the integrity of the vein wall from dilation may lead to long-term damage causing veins to remain dilated postpartum because of exposure to increased activity of matrix metalloproteinases (MMP) [66, 67]. The increase of MMP expression promotes the degradation of collagen, elastin, and endothelium, which directly impacts the ability of veins to control vascular wall tension [68]. The dilatation of pelvic veins can compress neighboring nerve bundles leading to pelvic pain [69].

Estrogen acts as a vasodilator and can induce vascular relaxation by stimulating prostacyclin and nitric oxide synthesis or by acting directly on the vascular smooth muscle to dilate the vessel [65, 70]. The hormonal changes that occur with pregnancy may also explain why the incidence of PCS increases as the number of pregnancies increases [71, 72].

Incompetent valves within the venous system result in retrograde venous flow or primary venous insufficiency. Borghi and Dell'Atti reported the incidence of ovarian vein valve incompetence in women of childbearing age being 35–46%. Secondary pelvic vein incompetence occurs due to a venous outflow obstruction [70]. This outflow obstruction is caused by extrinsic compression on the venous system, such as in left renal vein compression (nutcracker phenomenon), where the left renal vein is compressed between the abdominal aorta and superior mesenteric artery, or left iliac vein compression (May-Thurner), where the left common iliac vein is compressed by the right common iliac artery [73, 74]. The outflow obstruction prevents the venous system from draining leading to venous congestion. Venous overload can also occur from congenital or acquired malformations such as cirrhosis, tumor, or thrombus in the inferior vena cava, thrombus in the portal vein, or renal cell carcinoma with left renal vein thrombosis [75]. A less common venous outflow obstruction is caused by uterine malposition, which leads to ovarian vein compression, refluxing varicosities, and cross-pelvic venous collateral development causing painful venous congestion in the peroneal region [76].

Clinical Presentation

The American Vein and Lymphatic Society International Working Group on Pelvic Venous Disorders published a report with a Symptoms-Varices-Pathophysiology (SVP) classification in 2021 to define the variable clinical presentation as well as the underlying pathophysiology noting that vascular compressions may overlap [71]. Chronic pelvic pain has been reported to affect between 6 and 27% of women worldwide [77], and there is known association between chronic pelvic pain and the presence of dilated pelvic veins with pelvic venous insufficiency [61, 76]. Up to 60% of females with pelvic varicosities have symptoms of PCS [70, 78].

The symptoms associated with PCS arise from venous hypertension in the pelvis, which distends the peri-uterine plexus causing pain and pressure. Symptoms may include pelvic pain or pressure lasting for more than 6 months; pain exacerbated just prior to or during menses; pain with increased abdominal pressure (long periods of standing, walking, lifting) and alleviated with laying down; pain with coitus, during pregnancy, and with subsequent pregnancies; and the presence or history of vulvovaginal, gluteal, perineal, varicosities [76, 79].

Vulvar varicosities occur in 24–40% of patients with PCS [80]. These varicosities develop from the extensive venous reflux in the tributaries of the internal iliac veins, which transmit the pressure through the pelvic floor into the veins of the lower extremities [65, 81]. While PCS is a common cause of pelvic pain in females, affecting up to 40% of all females during one's lifetime, it is often misdiagnosed or underdiagnosed [76]. Pelvic pain is the chief complaint for up to 20% of gynecological visits annually [60].

Diagnosis

Once other pelvic pathologies have been ruled out, imaging to assess the pelvic veins for size, competence, and drainage is needed to diagnose PCS. Currently, there are no consistent diagnostic criteria for the diagnosis of PCS. The Society for Vascular Surgery (SVS) and the American Venous Forum (AVF) released clinical practice guidelines citing that premenopausal women presenting with varicose veins should be assessed for symptoms of PCS [82]. The first-line imaging study to screen for PCS is an ultrasound. Traditional ultrasonography can identify structural abnormalities or masses within the pelvis, while color-Doppler imaging can show the pelvic vasculature. Ultrasound can be useful to detect pelvic venous reflux and the measurement of pelvic vein diameters. PCS diagnosis is supported in cases with tortuous pelvic veins with a diameter greater than 4 mm, sluggish venous flow (3 cm/s), and dilated arcuate veins in the myometrium communicating with pelvic varicosities [83]. Gloviczki cited that an ovarian vein diameter greater than 6 mm seen on ultrasonography carries a 96% positive-predictive value for pelvic varices [82]. Steenbeek found that a pelvic vein greater than 5 mm, which crosses the uterine body, along with pelvic varicosities and reflux, were the most indicative findings of PCS seen on ultrasound [84].

Cross-sectional imaging, particularly CT venography and MRV, provides useful anatomic data in the diagnosis of PCS, particularly if the cause is related to a venous compression, such as May-Thurner or left renal vein compression [76]. The SVS and AVF clinical practice guidelines cite MR and CT as suitable methods to identify pelvic venous obstruction or iliac vein stenosis in patients with lower extremity varicosities when a proximal obstruction or compression is suspected [82]. Within the guidelines, an ovarian vein diameter >8 mm coupled with four or more tortuous pelvic veins or dilated veins >4 mm in diameter confirms the diagnosis [82]. Due to the supine positioning during CT and MR, these tests may underestimate venous pathology [70].

Venography is the gold standard for diagnosing PCS as it allows for direct examination of the ovarian and iliac veins [70, 76, 82] (Fig. 7.5). To improve the demonstration of varicosities, contrast media, positioning the patient in a semi-upright or reverse Trendelenburg position, and performing the Valsalva maneuver can aid in the detection of abnormal vein diameters and degree of reflux [70, 76]. The SVS and AVF clinical practice guidelines give a criterion for diagnosing PCS, which includes one or more of the following findings: an ovarian vein diameter ≥6 mm, contrast retention ≥20 s, congestion of the pelvic venous plexus, opacification of the ipsilateral (or contralateral) internal iliac vein, and filling of vulvovaginal and thigh varicosities [82, 85].

Venography is needed to confirm PCS prior to potential intervention [85]. Macher found that pretreatment imaging was often lacking and that patients with multiple potential sources of pelvic pain (endometriosis, pain syndromes, irritable

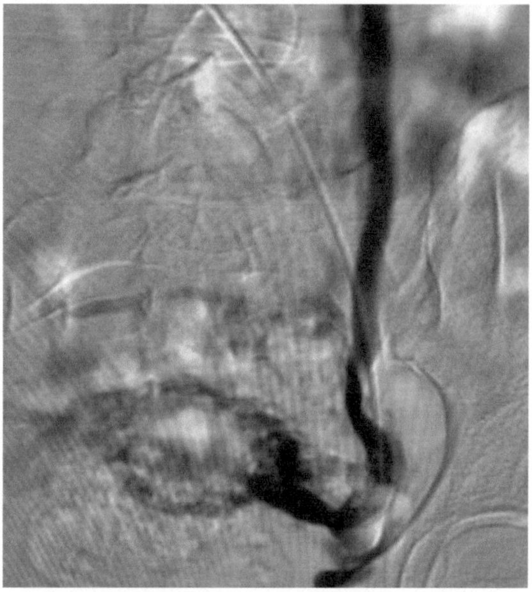

Fig. 7.5 Venogram demonstrating ovarian vein reflux (Photos courtesy of Dr. KH Nagarsheth MD)

bowel syndrome) may have a CT scan in their records alone prior to treatment [72]. Laparoscopy can also be used to exclude other pelvic pathologic conditions such as endometriosis. Laparoscopy is not useful in diagnosing incompetent veins due to supine positioning during the procedure and abdominal insufflation with carbon dioxide that may mask the refluxing veins [86].

Treatment

Medical management is the first-line treatment for PCS. Hormonal changes to the structure and elasticity of the pelvic venous system are known potential causes for PCS; hence, medical management centers around hormonal modulation. Hormonal agonists, such as progestogen, have been shown to be effective in reducing up to 50% of symptoms when compared to placebo with lasting effects, while women taking gonadotropin-releasing hormone modulators, such as goserelin, reported more improvement in overall pain when compared to progestogen [87]. Gonadotropin-releasing hormone agonists stabilize estrogen levels, which can aid in pain reduction [88]. Gabapentin has been used to treat neuropathic pain stemming from other medical conditions and has also been shown to improve pain intensity in women with PCS [89]. Additionally, gabapentin has been reported to have greater efficacy in pain reduction when compared to the off-label use of amitriptyline for its analgesic properties [90].

Targeted surgical treatment of PCS started in the 1980s in the form of extraperitoneal resection of the left ovarian vein to relieve the symptoms of PCS [91]. Hysterectomy was also a treatment option for chronic pelvic pain; however, a third of these patients never achieved pain relief and 20% had symptom recurrence [92]. In 1993, Edwards started performing surgical ligation of the ovarian veins with foam or an embolization agent based on the idea that PCS pain stems from venous reflux and incompetent ovarian veins [93].

Endovascular techniques aimed at decreasing blood flow through the gonadal veins have been shown to be safe and effective in treating PCS [94]. Embolization of incompetent ovarian veins has been shown to decrease pain and improve quality of life with minimal risk of complications from the procedure [86]. Pelvic vein embolization is the currently accepted treatment for PCS; however, this is based on empiric data and case reports rather than formal trials [70, 95]. Champaneria reported that 75% of patients found symptom relief after embolization of ovarian veins [96], which mirrors what other investigators found. Long-term symptom relief has been cited to occur in 70–90% of cases, where PCS is treated with ovarian vein embolization [97].

In cases where MTS is also present, treating the iliac vein compression can result in symptom relief without directly treating the pelvic veins. Endovascular stenting of the left iliac vein has been shown to be an effective technique for relieving symptoms of PCS with combined iliac vein compression [98]. One study found stenting of the left iliac vein alone relieves PCS symptoms in 16.6% of patients; however, stenting of the left CIV in combination with embolization of the gonadal veins eliminated PCS symptoms in 83.4% of patients [99]. Advances are being made in medical and surgical treatments for PCS; however, robust studies are needed regarding diagnosis, treatment, and long-term outcomes to better inform treatment.

Summary

Vascular compression syndromes such as nutcracker syndrome, May-Thurner syndrome, and pelvic congestion syndrome represent an array of compressive pathologies with unique but often overlapping symptoms. These vascular pathologies are often difficult to diagnose or, even worse, ignored by clinicians. Failure to recognize and treat these vascular pathologies can result in patients living with debilitating chronic pain. The diagnosis and treatment of these disorders have evolved considerably with the advent of better imaging modalities and endovascular surgical techniques. With vascular surgery advancing at a rapid pace, it is our hope that the diagnosis and treatment of these disorders will continue to improve as well as outcomes. Finally, clinicians should be cognizant of these concomitant syndromes when treating median arcuate ligament syndrome to better screen, identify, and treat patients with vascular compressive disorders.

References

1. He Y, Wu Z, Chen S, Tian L, Li D, Li M, Jin W, Zhang H. Nutcracker syndrome–how well do we know it? Urology. 2014;83(1):12–7. https://doi.org/10.1016/j.urology.2013.08.033.
2. de Schepper A. "Nutcracker" phenomenon of the renal vein and venous pathology of the left kidney. J Belg Radiol. 1972;55:507–11.
3. Kurklinsky AK, Rooke TW. Nutcracker phenomenon and nutcracker syndrome. Mayo Clin Proc. 2010;85(6):552–9. https://doi.org/10.4065/mcp.2009.0586.
4. Stubberud A, Cheema S, Tronvik E, Matharu M. Nutcracker syndrome mimicking new daily persistent headache: a case report. Cephalalgia. 2020;40(9):1008–11. https://doi.org/10.1177/0333102420918554.
5. Ali-El-Dein B, Osman Y, Shehab El-Din AB, El-Diasty T, Mansour O, Ghoneim MA. Anterior and posterior nutcracker syndrome: a report on 11 cases. Transplant Proc. 2003;35(2):851–3. https://doi.org/10.1016/s0041-1345(02)04026-5.
6. Shaper KR, Jackson JE, Williams G. The nutcracker syndrome: an uncommon cause of haematuria. Br J Urol. 1994;74(2):144–6. https://doi.org/10.1111/j.1464-410x.1994.tb16575.x.
7. Farina R, Foti PV, Pennisi I, Vasile T, Clemenza M, Rosa G, Crimi L, Catalano M, Vacirca F, Basile A. Vascular compression syndromes: a pictorial review. Ultrasonography. 2022;41(3):444–61. https://doi.org/10.14366/usg.21233.
8. Amato ACM, da Silva AEC, Bernal IM, de Oliveira JC, Di Paschoal Almeida Ribeiro M, Schinzari PS, Dos Santos RV. Combined nutcracker and Ehlers-Danlos syndromes: a case report. EJVES Vasc Forum. 2020;47:12–7. https://doi.org/10.1016/j.ejvsvf.2020.02.005.
9. Dunphy L, Penna M, Tam E, El-Kafsi J. Left renal vein entrapment syndrome: nutcracker syndrome! BMJ Case Rep. 2019;12(9):e230877. https://doi.org/10.1136/bcr-2019-230877.
10. Shin JI, Park JM, Lee SM, Shin YH, Kim JH, Lee JS, Kim MJ. Factors affecting spontaneous resolution of hematuria in childhood nutcracker syndrome. Pediatr Nephrol. 2005;20(5):609–13. https://doi.org/10.1007/s00467-004-1799-z.
11. Karaosmanoğlu D, Karcaaltincaba M, Akata D, Ozmen M. Unusual causes of left renal vein compression along its course: MDCT findings in patients with nutcracker and pelvic congestion syndrome. Surg Radiol Anat. 2010;32(4):323–7. https://doi.org/10.1007/s00276-009-0548-1.
12. Scultetus AH, Villavicencio JL, Gillespie DL. The nutcracker syndrome: its role in the pelvic venous disorders. J Vasc Surg. 2001;34(5):812–9. https://doi.org/10.1067/mva.2001.118802.
13. Inal M, Unal Daphan B, Karadeniz Bilgili MY. Superior mesenteric artery syndrome accompanying with nutcracker syndrome: a case report. Iran Red Crescent Med J. 2014;16(10):e14755. https://doi.org/10.5812/ircmj.14755.
14. Laskowski T, Tihonov N, Richard M, et al. Concurrent nutcracker syndrome and superior mesenteric artery syndrome requiring duodenojejunal bypass and left renal vein transposition. Ann Vasc Surg. 2022;2:100099. https://doi.org/10.1016/j.avsurg.2022.100099.
15. Daily R, Matteo J, Loper T, Northup M. Nutcracker syndrome: symptoms of syncope and hypotension improved following endovascular stenting. Vascular. 2012;20(6):337–41. https://doi.org/10.1258/vasc.2011.
16. Shin JI, Park JM, Lee JS, Kim MJ. Effect of renal Doppler ultrasound on the detection of nutcracker syndrome in children with hematuria. Eur J Pediatr. 2007;166(5):399–404. https://doi.org/10.1007/s00431-006-0252-7.
17. Calado R, Braz M, Lobo L, Simão C. Nutcracker syndrome. Hematuria without diagnosis? Acta Medica Port. 2011;24(3):695–8.
18. Kim SH. Doppler US and CT diagnosis of nutcracker syndrome. Korean J Radiol. 2019;20(12):1627–37. https://doi.org/10.3348/kjr.2019.0084.
19. Kolber MK, Cui Z, Chen CK, Habibollahi P, Kalva SP. Nutcracker syndrome: diagnosis and therapy. Cardiovasc Diagn Ther. 2021;11(5):1140–9. https://doi.org/10.21037/cdt-20-160.
20. Avgerinos ED, McEnaney R, Chaer RA. Surgical and endovascular interventions for nutcracker syndrome. Semin Vasc Surg. 2013;26(4):170–7. https://doi.org/10.1053/j.semvascsurg.2014.06.014.

21. de Macedo GL, Dos Santos MA, Sarris AB, Gomes RZ. Diagnosis and treatment of the Nutcracker syndrome: a review of the last 10 years. J Vasc Bras. 2018;17(3):220–8. https://doi.org/10.1590/1677-5449.012417.
22. Ananthan K, Onida S, Davies AH. Nutcracker syndrome: an update on current diagnostic criteria and management guidelines. Eur J Vasc Endovasc Surg. 2017;53(6):886–94. https://doi.org/10.1016/j.ejvs.2017.02.015.
23. Hulsberg PC, McLoney E, Partovi S, Davidson JC, Patel IJ. Minimally invasive treatments for venous compression syndromes. Cardiovasc Diagn Ther. 2016;6(6):582–92. https://doi.org/10.21037/cdt.2016.10.01.
24. Said SM, Gloviczki P, Kalra M, Oderich GS, Duncan AA, Fleming M, Bower TC. Renal nutcracker syndrome: surgical options. Semin Vasc Surg. 2013;26(1):35–42. https://doi.org/10.1053/j.semvascsurg.2013.04.006.
25. Menard MT. Nutcracker syndrome: when should it be treated and how? Perspect Vasc Surg Endovasc Ther. 2009;21(2):117–24. https://doi.org/10.1177/1531003509338402.
26. Reed NR, Kalra M, Bower TC, Vrtiska TJ, Ricotta JJ, Gloviczki P. Left renal vein transposition for nutcracker syndrome. J Vasc Surg. 2009;49(2):386–93. https://doi.org/10.1016/j.jvs.2008.09.051.
27. Wang L, Yi L, Yang L, Liu Z, Rao J, Liu L, Yang J. Diagnosis and surgical treatment of nutcracker syndrome: a single-center experience. Urology. 2009;73(4):871–6. https://doi.org/10.1016/j.urology.2008.11.043.
28. Liu Y, Sun Y, Jin X. Left renocaval venous bypass with autologous great saphenous vein for nutcracker syndrome. J Vasc Surg. 2012;55(5):1482–4. https://doi.org/10.1016/j.jvs.2011.08.053.
29. Chen S, Zhang H, Shi H, Tian L, Jin W, Li M. Endovascular stenting for treatment of Nutcracker syndrome: report of 61 cases with long-term followup. J Urol. 2011;186(2):570–5. https://doi.org/10.1016/j.juro.2011.03.135.
30. Perkov D, Vrkić Kirhmajer M, Novosel L, Popić RJ. Transcatheter ovarian vein embolisation without renal vein stenting for pelvic venous congestion and nutcracker anatomy. Vasa. 2016;45(4):337–41. https://doi.org/10.1024/0301-1526/a000547.
31. Virchow R. Ueber die Erweiterung kleinerer Gefäfse. Archiv Pathol Anat. 1851;3:427–62. https://doi.org/10.1007/BF01960918.
32. May R, Thurner J. The cause of the predominantly sinistral occurrence of thrombosis of the pelvic veins. Angiology. 1957;8(5):419–27. https://doi.org/10.1177/000331975700800505.
33. Cockett FB, Thomas ML. The iliac compression syndrome. Br J Surg. 1965;52(10):816–21. https://doi.org/10.1002/bjs.1800521028.
34. Knuttinen MG, Naidu S, Oklu R, Kriegshauser S, Eversman W, Rotellini L, Thorpe PE. May-Thurner: diagnosis and endovascular management. Cardiovasc Diagn Ther. 2017;7(Suppl 3):S159–64. https://doi.org/10.21037/cdt.2017.10.14.
35. Brinegar KN, Sheth RA, Khademhosseini A, Bautista J, Oklu R. Iliac vein compression syndrome: clinical, imaging and pathologic findings. World J Radiol. 2015;7(11):375–81. https://doi.org/10.4329/wjr.v7.i11.375.
36. Yi JA, Hadley JB, Kuwayama DP. Atypical May-Thurner syndrome caused by endovascular aortic aneurysm repair. J Vasc Surg Cases Innov Tech. 2020;6(3):397–400. https://doi.org/10.1016/j.jvscit.2020.06.004.
37. Raju S, Neglen P. High prevalence of nonthrombotic iliac vein lesions in chronic venous disease: a permissive role in pathogenicity. J Vasc Surg. 2006;44(1):136–43. https://doi.org/10.1016/j.jvs.2006.02.065.
38. Kaltenmeier CT, Erben Y, Indes J, Lee A, Dardik A, Sarac T, Ochoa Chaar CI. Systematic review of May-Thurner syndrome with emphasis on gender differences. J Vasc Surg Venous Lymphat Disord. 2018;6(3):399–407. https://doi.org/10.1016/j.jvsv.2017.11.006.
39. Barry A. Sonography's role in the diagnosis of May-Thurner syndrome. J Diagn Med Sonogr. 2018;34(1):65–70. https://doi.org/10.1177/8756479317714796.

40. Lugo-Fagundo C, Nance JW, Johnson PT, Fishman EK. May-Thurner syndrome: MDCT findings and clinical correlates. Abdom Radiol. 2016;41(10):2026–30. https://doi.org/10.1007/s00261-016-0793-9.
41. Ibrahim W, Al Safran Z, Hasan H, Zeid WA. Endovascular management of May-Thurner syndrome. Ann Vasc Dis. 2012;5(2):217–21. https://doi.org/10.3400/avd.cr.12.00007.
42. Heller T, Teichert C, Hafer J, Weber MA, Kröger JC, Meinel FG. Prevalence of May-Thurner syndrome in patients with deep vein thrombosis at a large medical referral center. Röfo. 2019;191(12):1107–17. https://doi.org/10.1055/a-0959-6230.
43. Kibbe MR, Ujiki M, Goodwin AL, Eskandari M, Yao J, Matsumura J. Iliac vein compression in an asymptomatic patient population. J Vasc Surg. 2004;39(5):937–43. https://doi.org/10.1016/j.jvs.2003.12.032.
44. Rohr A, Maxwell K, Best S, Lemons S, Johnson P. Rare presentation and endovascular treatment of multifocal iliac venous stenoses due to right sided May-Thurner syndrome. Radiol Case Rep. 2019;15(3):201–3. https://doi.org/10.1016/j.radcr.2019.11.013.
45. Dunlap E, Fitzpatrick S, Nagarsheth K. Back pain and right leg swelling: unusual presentations of May-Thurner syndrome. Cureus. 2023;15(3):e35984. https://doi.org/10.7759/cureus.35984.
46. Suwanabol PA, Tefera G, Schwarze ML. Syndromes associated with the deep veins: phlegmasia cerulea dolens, May-Thurner syndrome, and nutcracker syndrome. Perspect Vasc Surg Endovasc Ther. 2010;22(4):223–30. https://doi.org/10.1177/1531003511400426.
47. Mousa AY, AbuRahma AF. May-Thurner syndrome: update and review. Ann Vasc Surg. 2013;27(7):984–95. https://doi.org/10.1016/j.avsg.2013.05.001.
48. Lamba R, Tanner DT, Sekhon S, McGahan JP, Corwin MT, Lall CG. Multidetector CT of vascular compression syndromes in the abdomen and pelvis. Radiographics. 2014;34(1):93–115. https://doi.org/10.1148/rg.341125010.
49. Farina R, Foti PV, Iannace FA, Fanzone L, Pennisi I, Conti A, Santonocito S, Basile A. May Thurner syndrome: description of a case with unusual clinical onset. J Ultrasound. 2022;25(2):309–13. https://doi.org/10.1007/s40477-020-00497-0.
50. Liu Z, Gao N, Shen L, Yang J, Zhu Y, Li Z, Si Y. Endovascular treatment for symptomatic iliac vein compression syndrome: a prospective consecutive series of 48 patients. Ann Vasc Surg. 2014;28(3):695–704. https://doi.org/10.1016/j.avsg.2013.05.019.
51. Hsu YC, Huang YK, Hsu LS, Chen PY, Chen CW. Using non-contrast-enhanced magnetic resonance venography for the evaluation of May-Thurner syndrome in patients with renal insufficiency: a case report. Medicine. 2019;98(52):e18427. https://doi.org/10.1097/MD.0000000000018427.
52. Zucker EJ, Ganguli S, Ghoshhajra BB, Gupta R, Prabhakar AM. Imaging of venous compression syndromes. Cardiovasc Diagn Ther. 2016;6(6):519–32. https://doi.org/10.21037/cdt.2016.11.19.
53. Forauer AR, Gemmete JJ, Dasika NL, Cho KJ, Williams DM. Intravascular ultrasound in the diagnosis and treatment of iliac vein compression (May-Thurner) syndrome. J Vasc Interv Radiol. 2002;13(5):523–7. https://doi.org/10.1016/s1051-0443(07)61535-8.
54. Radaideh Q, Patel NM, Shammas NW. Iliac vein compression: epidemiology, diagnosis and treatment. Vasc Health Risk Manag. 2019;15:115–22. https://doi.org/10.2147/VHRM.S203349.
55. Poyyamoli S, Mehta P, Cherian M, Anand RR, Patil SB, Kalva S, Salazar G. May-Thurner syndrome. Cardiovasc Diagn Ther. 2021;11(5):1104–11. https://doi.org/10.21037/cdt.2020.03.07.
56. Bi Y, Yu Z, Chen H, Ren J, Han X. Long-term outcome and quality of life in patients with iliac vein compression syndrome after endovascular treatment. Phlebology. 2019;34(8):536–42. https://doi.org/10.1177/0268355518825090.
57. Oğuzkurt L, Ozkan U, Tercan F, Koç Z. Ultrasonographic diagnosis of iliac vein compression (May-Thurner) syndrome. Diagn Interv Radiol. 2007;13(3):152–5.
58. Harbin MM, Lutsey PL. May-Thurner syndrome: history of understanding and need for defining population prevalence. J Thromb Haemost. 2020;18(3):534–42. https://doi.org/10.1111/jth.14707.

59. Behzadi AH, Khilnani NM, Zhang W, Bares AJ, Boddu SR, Min RJ, Prince MR. Pelvic cardiovascular magnetic resonance venography: venous changes with patient position and hydration status. J Cardiovasc Magn Reson. 2019;21(1):3. https://doi.org/10.1186/s12968-018-0503-6.
60. Koo S, Fan CM. Pelvic congestion syndrome and pelvic varicosities. Tech Vasc Interv Radiol. 2014;17(2):90–5. https://doi.org/10.1053/j.tvir.2014.02.005.
61. Jurga-Karwacka A, Karwacki GM, Schoetzau A, Zech CJ, Heinzelmann-Schwarz V, Schwab FD. A forgotten disease: pelvic congestion syndrome as a cause of chronic lower abdominal pain. PLoS One. 2019;14(4):e0213834. https://doi.org/10.1371/journal.pone.0213834.
62. Richet MA. Traité pratique d'anatomie médico-chirurgicale. E Chaamerot. Paris: Libraairee Editeur; 1857.
63. Chidekel N. Female pelvic veins demonstrated by selective renal phlebography with particular reference to pelvic varicosities. Acta Radiol Diagn. 1968;7(3):193–211. https://doi.org/10.1177/028418516800700301.
64. Bałabuszek K, Toborek M, Pietura R. Comprehensive overview of the venous disorder known as pelvic congestion syndrome. Ann Med. 2022;54(1):22–36. https://doi.org/10.1080/07853890.2021.2014556.
65. Mahmoud O, Vikatmaa P, Aho P, et al. Efficacy of endovascular treatment for pelvic congestion syndrome. J Vasc Surg Venous Lymphat Disord. 2016;4(3):355–70. https://doi.org/10.1016/j.jvsv.2016.01.002.
66. Kucukguven A, Khalil RA. Matrix metalloproteinases as potential targets in the venous dilation associated with varicose veins. Curr Drug Targets. 2013;14(3):287–324.
67. Szary C, Wilczko J, Plucinska D, et al. The number of pregnancies and deliveries and their association with selected morphological and hemodynamic parameters of the pelvic and abdominal venous system. J Clin Med. 2021;10(4):736. https://doi.org/10.3390/jcm10040736.
68. MacColl E, Khalil RA. Matrix metalloproteinases as regulators of vein structure and function: implications in chronic venous disease. J Pharmacol Exp Ther. 2015;355(3):410–28. https://doi.org/10.1124/jpet.115.227330.
69. Knuttinen MG, Xie K, Jani A, Palumbo A, Carrillo T, Mar W. Pelvic venous insufficiency: imaging diagnosis, treatment approaches, and therapeutic issues. AJR Am J Roentgenol. 2015;204(2):448–58. https://doi.org/10.2214/AJR.14.12709.
70. Borghi C, Dell'Atti L. Pelvic congestion syndrome: the current state of the literature. Arch Gynecol Obstet. 2016;293(2):291–301. https://doi.org/10.1007/s00404-015-3895-7.
71. Meissner MH, Khilnani NM, Labropoulos N, Gasparis AP, Gibson K, Greiner M, Learman LA, Atashroo D, Lurie F, Passman MA, Basile A, Lazarshvilli Z, Lohr J, Kim MD, Nicolini PH, Pabon-Ramos WM, Rosenblatt M. The symptoms-varices-pathophysiology classification of pelvic venous disorders: a report of the American Vein & Lymphatic Society International Working Group on pelvic venous disorders. J Vasc Surg Venous Lymphat Disord. 2021;9(3):568–84. https://doi.org/10.1016/j.jvsv.2020.12.084.
72. Macher J, Brahmbhatt A, Shetty A, Chughtai K, Baran T, Baah NO, Dogra V. Predicting pelvic congestion syndrome: Concomitant pelvic pain diagnoses do not affect venography or embolization outcomes. J Clin Imaging Sci. 2021;11:61. https://doi.org/10.25259/JCIS_180_2021.
73. Gulleroglu K, Gulleroglu B, Baskin E. Nutcracker syndrome. World J Nephrol. 2014;3(4):277–81. https://doi.org/10.5527/wjn.v3.i4.277.
74. Winer AG, Chakiryan NH, Mooney RP, Verges D, Ghanaat M, Allaei A, Robinson L, Zinn H, Lang EK. Secondary pelvic congestion syndrome: description and radiographic diagnosis. Can J Urol. 2014;21(4):7365–8.
75. Birn J, Vedantham S. May-Thurner syndrome and other obstructive iliac vein lesions: meaning, myth, and mystery. Vasc Med. 2015;20(1):74–83. https://doi.org/10.1177/1358863X14560429.
76. O'Brien MT, Gillespie DL. Diagnosis and treatment of the pelvic congestion syndrome. J Vasc Surg Venous Lymphat Disord. 2015;3(1):96–106. https://doi.org/10.1016/j.jvsv.2014.05.00.
77. Ahangari A. Prevalence of chronic pelvic pain among women: an updated review. Pain Physician. 2014;17(2):E141–7.

78. Daniels J, Gray R, Hills RK, et al. Laparoscopic uterosacral nerve ablation for alleviating chronic pelvic pain: a randomized controlled trial. JAMA. 2009;302(9):955–61. https://doi.org/10.1001/jama.2009.1268.
79. Asciutto G, Asciutto KC, Mumme A, Geier B. Pelvic venous incompetence: reflux patterns and treatment results. Eur J Vasc Endovasc Surg. 2009;38(3):381–6. https://doi.org/10.1016/j.ejvs.2009.05.023.
80. Kim AS, Greyling LA, Davis LS. Vulvar varicosities: a review. Dermatologic Surg. 2017;43(3):351–6. https://doi.org/10.1097/DSS.0000000000001008.
81. Bendek B, Afuape N, Banks E, Desai NA. Comprehensive review of pelvic congestion syndrome: causes, symptoms, treatment options. Curr Opin Obstet Gynecol. 2020;32(4):237–42. https://doi.org/10.1097/GCO.0000000000000637.
82. Gloviczki P, Comerota AJ, Dalsing MC, Eklof BG, Gillespie DL, Gloviczki ML, Lohr JM, McLafferty RB, Meissner MH, Murad MH, Padberg FT, Pappas PJ, Passman MA, Raffetto JD, Vasquez MA, Wakefield TW, Society for Vascular Surgery; American Venous Forum. The care of patients with varicose veins and associated chronic venous diseases: clinical practice guidelines of the Society for Vascular Surgery and the American Venous Forum. J Vasc Surg. 2011;53(5 Suppl):2S–48S. https://doi.org/10.1016/j.jvs.2011.01.079.
83. Patel MD, Young SW, Dahiya N. Ultrasound of pelvic pain in the nonpregnant woman. Radiol Clin North Am. 2019;57(3):601–16. https://doi.org/10.1016/j.rcl.2019.01.010.
84. Steenbeek MP, van der Vleuten CJM, Schultze Kool LJ, Nieboer TE. Noninvasive diagnostic tools for pelvic congestion syndrome: a systematic review. Acta Obstet Gynecol Scand. 2018;97(7):776–86. https://doi.org/10.1111/aogs.13311.
85. Arnoldussen CW, de Wolf MA, Wittens CH. Diagnostic imaging of pelvic congestive syndrome. Phlebology. 2015;30(Suppl):67–72.
86. Dorobisz TA, Garcarek JS, Kurcz J, et al. Diagnosis and treatment of pelvic congestion syndrome: single-centre experiences. Adv Clin Exp Med. 2017;26(2):269–76. https://doi.org/10.17219/acem/68158.
87. Cheong YC, Smotra G, Williams AC. Non-surgical interventions for the management of chronic pelvic pain. Cochrane Database Syst Rev. 2014;3:CD008797. https://doi.org/10.1002/14651858.CD008797.pub2.
88. Resta C, Moustogiannis A, Chatzinikita E, et al. Gonadotropin-releasing hormone (GnRH)/GnRH receptors and their role in the treatment of endometriosis. Cureus. 2023;15(4):e38136. https://doi.org/10.7759/cureus.38136.
89. Fan XM, Ren YF, Fu X, et al. Gabapentin has longer-term efficacy for the treatment of chronic pelvic pain in women: a systematic review and pilot meta-analysis. Pain Ther. 2021;10(2):1673–89. https://doi.org/10.1007/s40122-021-00330-4.
90. Lewis SC, Bhattacharya S, Wu O, Vincent K, Jack SA, Critchley HO, Porter MA, Cranley D, Wilson JA, Horne AW. Gabapentin for the management of chronic pelvic pain in women (GaPP1): a pilot randomised controlled trial. PLoS One. 2016;11(4):e0153037. https://doi.org/10.1371/journal.pone.0153037.
91. Rundqvist E, Sandholm LE, Larsson G. Treatment of pelvic varicosities causing lower abdominal pain with extraperitoneal resection of the left ovarian vein. Ann Chir Gynaecol. 1984;73(6):339–41.
92. Beard RW, Kennedy RG, Gangar KF, Stones RW, Rogers V, Reginald PW, Anderson M. Bilateral oophorectomy and hysterectomy in the treatment of intractable pelvic pain associated with pelvic congestion. Br J Obstet Gynaecol. 1991;98(10):988–92. https://doi.org/10.1111/j.1471-0528.1991.tb15336.x.
93. Edwards RD, Robertson IR, MacLean AB, Hemingway AP. Case report: pelvic pain syndrome–successful treatment of a case by ovarian vein embolization. Clin Radiol. 1993;47(6):429–31. https://doi.org/10.1016/s0009-9260(05)81067-0.
94. Gavrilov SG, Sazhin A, Krasavin G, Moskalenko E, Mishakina N. Comparative analysis of the efficacy and safety of endovascular and endoscopic interventions on the gonadal

veins in the treatment of pelvic congestion syndrome. J Vasc Surg Venous Lymphat Disord. 2021;9(1):178–86. https://doi.org/10.1016/j.jvsv.2020.05.013.
95. Daniels JP, Champaneria R, Shah L, Gupta JK, Birch J, Moss JG. Effectiveness of embolization or sclerotherapy of pelvic veins for reducing chronic pelvic pain: a systematic review. J Vasc Interv Radiol. 2016;27(10):1478–86. https://doi.org/10.1016/j.jvir.2016.04.016.
96. Champaneria R, Shah L, Moss J, Gupta JK, Birch J, Middleton LJ, Daniels JP. The relationship between pelvic vein incompetence and chronic pelvic pain in women: systematic reviews of diagnosis and treatment effectiveness. Health Technol Assess. 2016;20(5):1–108. https://doi.org/10.3310/hta20050.
97. Kashef E, Evans E, Patel N, Agrawal D, Hemingway AP. Pelvic venous congestion syndrome: female venous congestive syndromes and endovascular treatment options. CVIR Endovasc. 2023;6(1):25. https://doi.org/10.1186/s42155-023-00365-y.
98. Yetkin E, Ozturk S, Cuglan B, Turhan H. Symptoms in dilating venous disease. Curr Cardiol Rev. 2020;16(3):164–72. https://doi.org/10.2174/1573403X16666200312101245.
99. Gavrilov SG, Vasilyev AV, Krasavin GV, Moskalenko YP, Mishakina NY. Endovascular interventions in the treatment of pelvic congestion syndrome caused by May-Thurner syndrome. J Vasc Surg Venous Lymphat Disord. 2020;8(6):1049–57. https://doi.org/10.1016/j.jvsv.2020.02.012.

Chapter 8
Gastrointestinal Compression Associated with Median Arcuate Ligament Syndrome: Superior Mesenteric Artery Syndrome

Gabriela Lozano, Eleanor Dunlap, Khanjan H. Nagarsheth, and Daniel Shouhed

Introduction

Superior mesenteric artery syndrome (SMAS) is defined as compression of the third portion of the duodenum between the aorta and the superior mesenteric artery. It was first described by Carl Freiherr von Rokitansky in 1842 as the entrapment and obstruction of the third portion of the duodenum [1, 2]. SMAS was further described by Wilkie in 1921, but it was not until 1927 that he published the first large case series including 75 patients. Soon after, SMAS was widely recognized as Wilkie's syndrome [3]. Based on his research, Wilkie also concluded that the treatment of choice for SMAS should be a duodenojejunostomy. In 1908, the first operation for SMAS was performed at Johns Hopkins involving a duodenojejunostomy [4]. SMAS has also become known as duodenal compression syndrome, arteriomesenteric duodenal obstruction, chronic duodenal ileus, and cast syndrome [3–6].

SMAS is exceedingly rare with a reported incidence of 0.013–0.3%, with many reports limited to case reports and small case series [1, 3, 6, 7]. SMAS is more commonly found in young adults between the ages of 10 and 39. Two-thirds of afflicted patients are female, and eighty percent of patients have an asthenic body habitus [8, 9]. However, it is important to note this can also occur in males and affect patients of any age. While familial cases have been reported in the literature there does not appear to be an ethnic or racial predisposition [9].

G. Lozano · D. Shouhed (✉)
Robotic Surgical Institute of Southern California, Beverly Hills, CA, USA

E. Dunlap · K. H. Nagarsheth
Division of Vascular Surgery, Department of Surgery, University of Maryland, Baltimore, MD, USA

D. Shouhed et al. (eds.), *Median Arcuate Ligament Syndrome*,
https://doi.org/10.1007/978-3-031-80740-4_8

Etiology

SMAS is characterized by extrinsic compression of the third portion of the duodenum between the superior mesenteric artery and the aorta, leading to a complete or partial duodenal outlet obstruction [10]. This compression is often caused by a decrease of the intervening mesenteric fat pad between the aorta and SMA, which in turn leads to a decrease of the aortomesenteric angle and aortomesenteric distance below normal values (Fig. 8.1). The mesenteric fat pad between the SMA and the duodenum serves the function of holding the SMA off the spine, thus preventing compression of the duodenum. Loss of this intervening fat pad makes the duodenum more vulnerable to compression between the SMA and the aorta. Normally, the aortomesenteric angle is 45°, often ranging from 25 to 65°, producing a normal aortomesenteric distance that ranges from 10 to 28 mm [3, 5, 11, 12]. Reduction of the aortomesenteric angle below 25° will lead to a diminished aortomesenteric distance and may cause compression of the third portion of the duodenum [9, 11] (Fig. 8.2).

The etiology of SMAS is often divided into two categories: congenital and acquired causes. Congenital causes are often linked to anatomical variants in a subset of patients, such as a short mesenteric root, a high retroperitoneal attachment of the ligament of Treitz, and/or a low origin of the SMA [3]. SMA syndrome is often secondary to another condition leading to rapid or profound weight loss. Weight loss can be attributed to a variety of factors, including severe and debilitating illness or wasting diseases, eating disorders, traumatic injury, malabsorption syndromes, postoperative states—including bariatric surgery, esophagectomy, and abdominal trauma [1, 3]. Narrowing of the aortomesenteric angle and aortomesenteric distance can also be seen in patients who develop SMA syndrome as a result of corrective

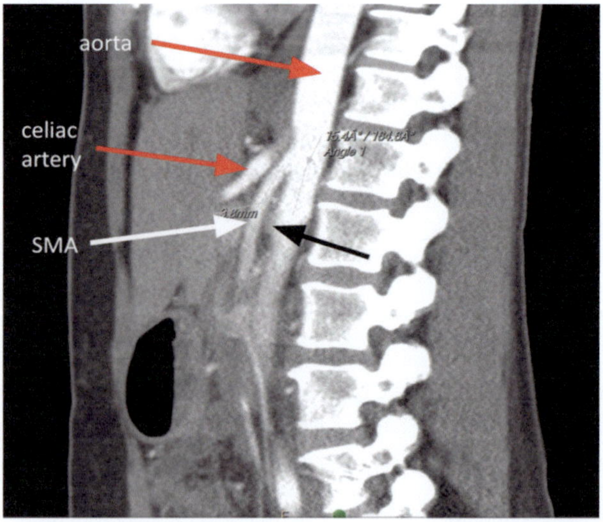

Fig. 8.1 Sagittal view showing compression of the duodenum (black arrow) by the superior mesenteric artery. Aortomesenteric angle of 15°, aortomesenteric distance of 3.8 mm

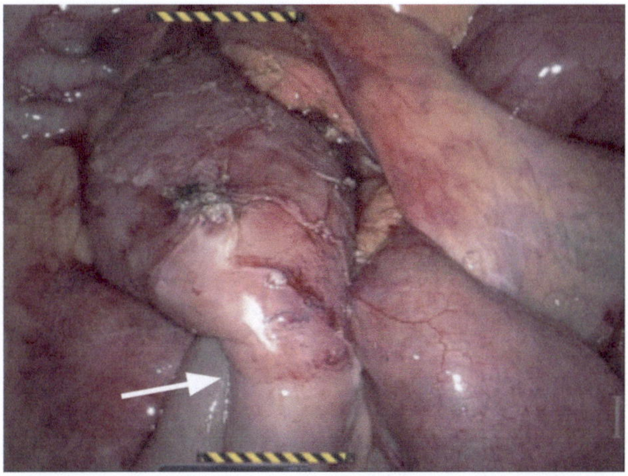

Fig. 8.2 Dilatation proximal to the region of obstruction after duodenal derotation. The white arrow highlights the area of compression by the SMA at the junction between the 3rd and 4th portions of the duodenum

surgery for scoliosis. In this setting, the condition arises as the relative lengthening of the spine after surgery increases the tension of the mesentery causing narrowing of the aortomesenteric angle and distance. When this compression is developed after surgical treatment for spinal deformities, it is known as cast syndrome [13].

The biggest risk factor for SMAS is significant weight loss, which is not uncommon in the setting of MALS. Notably, we have observed that SMAS may develop in as many as 23% of patients with MALS, typically arising after profound weight loss due to the severe debilitating nature of postprandial pain caused by MALS. Additionally, in 2021, Sandmann et al. documented a series of 122 patients who underwent open vascular surgery for an array of vascular compressions, and 31% of patients were documented to have undergone surgery for both MALS and SMAS. It is our practice to always investigate the primary etiology of SMAS; however, Akin et al. note that up to 40.4% of SMAS cases have no apparent etiology [14].

Clinical Presentation

Symptoms of SMAS are often similar to those of small bowel or gastric outlet obstruction [7]. Typical symptoms of SMAS include a feeling of epigastric fullness, postprandial nausea, intermittent or chronic emesis, and abdominal pain [11, 15, 16]. It is noted that abdominal pain, vomiting, early satiety, and nausea are often the most common symptoms, though patients may present with a constellation of symptoms [7]. Patients often present with a long history of chronic abdominal complaints and presentation can vary depending on the etiology and degree of duodenal compression. Patients who have undergone surgery for scoliosis often exhibit symptoms within the first postoperative week [17]. Furthermore, the severity of symptoms often varies with the degree of compression. Patients with severe compression, or total obstruction, often present with severe nausea, bilious emesis of partially undigested food, and abdominal distention [3].

As mentioned previously, SMAS can be a secondary condition seen in the setting of MALS. Much of the available literature denotes that epigastric abdominal pain is often the chief complaint of patients presenting with SMAS [1, 3, 7]. However, we have observed that epigastric postprandial pain with acute onset is a typical feature of MALS. Postprandial abdominal pain that is a result of SMAS is primarily localized to the periumbilical region and is cramping in nature, with an onset time later than that of MALS. Furthermore, patients in our practice have noted that these are two distinct pains often with different intensities. A classic feature of MALS is postprandial abdominal pain exacerbated by all foods and liquids, whereas postprandial pain seen in the setting of SMAS is often aggravated by tough, chewy, and fibrous foods, such as legumes, chicken breast, and steak.

A key differentiating feature of abdominal pain caused by MALS is the fact that it is often alleviated by a celiac nerve block. A celiac ganglion nerve block can be used for both diagnostic and therapeutic purposes as patients with MALS often experience significant, profound relief of postprandial pain after the block. Consequently, patients with a component of SMAS may report continued periumbilical pain and often experience continued postprandial nausea and/or vomiting.

The presentation of patients with SMAS closely resembles that of patients with gastroparesis. Symptoms of gastroparesis include nausea, vomiting, early satiety, bloating, postprandial fullness, abdominal pain, and weight loss [18]. Additionally, patients also report intolerance to fibrous, chewy foods much like that seen in patients with SMAS. A full workup consisting of a 4-hour gastric emptying scan is necessary to rule out gastroparesis as a possible contributing factor to the patient's picture.

Diagnosis

SMA Syndrome is a diagnosis that requires a considerably high index of suspicion as this compression syndrome presents with vague symptoms of bowel obstruction and can be attributed to other causes [5]. It is important that patients suspected of having SMAS undergo a thorough workup to rule out any other potential etiology and clearly ascertain a diagnosis [3]. Upper gastrointestinal series, CT or MR angiography, ultrasonography, and endoscopy can all be used for establishing a diagnosis [17]. Rather than serving in clinching a diagnosis, endoscopy can be useful in investigating other possible complications associated with a proximal small bowel obstruction, including biliary reflux, gastritis, and duodenal ulcers. Endoscopy may also serve to rule out other causes of duodenal compression [9].

CT angiography is an exceptionally useful diagnostic tool as it allows for accurate measurement of the aortomesenteric angle and aortomesenteric distance [9] (Fig. 8.1). An aortomesenteric angle of <22–25° and an aortomesenteric distance of <8 mm have exhibited a strong correlation with symptoms of SMAS. Furthermore, an aortomesenteric angle of <25° is regarded as being the

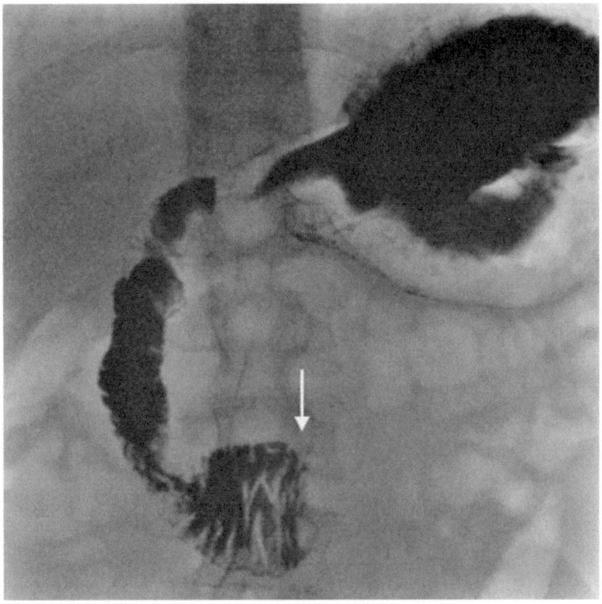

Fig. 8.3 This UGI demonstrates compression of the third part of the duodenum and an abrupt cut-off of contrast to the left of the arrow

most sensitive measure of diagnosis, especially if observed in the setting of an aortomesenteric distance <8 mm. These cutoff measurements have been cited to be highly specific for at least one symptom of SMAS [1, 19].

While an upper GI series plays an important role in diagnosis, CT and MR angiography are favored due to their high specificity and sensitivity. An UGI series is not highly sensitive as liquids may be observed passing through the region of obstruction where solids would typically not pass through. Classic upper GI findings in the setting of SMAS are dilatation of the first and second portions of the duodenum, occlusion, and tapering of contrast as it passes through the region of obstruction, to-and-fro motion, delayed contrast transit time, or an abrupt vertical or oblique compression of the third portion of the duodenum [4, 5, 15, 17] (Fig. 8.3).

Radiographic imaging findings alone are not sufficient in diagnosing SMA syndrome. A significant positive correlation has been found between diminished aortomesenteric distance and low BMI [12]. As such, these imaging findings must be placed in the appropriate clinical context as reduced aortomesenteric angles and distances may be observed in individuals without correlating compressive symptoms.

Treatment

Various treatment options have been proposed for SMAS. Much of the literature claims that the key to the resolution of symptoms lies in the reversal of weight loss promoting the restoration of the mesenteric fat pad, thereby leading to an increase of the narrowed aortomesenteric angle and distance [3]. As such, conservative medical management is often the first course of treatment for SMAS. This may include fluid resuscitation, bowel rest, and total parenteral nutrition. Hyperalimentation with the use of a nasojejunal or gastrojejunal feeding tube inserted past the region of obstruction is also recommended and is quoted to have a 70% chance of improvement, especially in an acute setting [17]. Hyperalimentation is quoted to have a particularly high success rate in patients with a short history of symptoms. In the case of patients with long-term, chronic symptoms, conservative treatment often involves a prolonged hospital stay and is correlated with a low success rate [1]. In this case, a patient may be quoted to have a 14–75% chance of improvement [6, 8]. In our experience, and in the experience of Dr. Domingo Alvear, hyperalimentation and conservative management have not been successful in improving symptoms. It is speculated that while a patient can regain weight, the compressed region of bowel has developed a stricture which remains even if the aortomesenteric angle and distance has increased. Furthermore, guidelines for the length of medical management have not been established, though Ganss et al. recommend a trial of medical management under 3 months to prevent disease chronicity and progression [5].

Surgical treatment is indicated in symptomatic patients who fail to experience improvement from conservative treatment. Sun et al. also reported that an aggressive surgical approach is warranted when the diagnosis of SMAS is both clinically and radiologically clear. This is based on the assumption that surgical intervention may lead to the complete resolution of symptoms and allow the patient to resume oral feeding. However, it is noted that this may not always be the case [5, 6]. Several surgical procedures including gastrojejunostomy, the Strong procedure, duodenal derotation, and duodenojejunostomy (DDJ) have been proposed [8, 17]. Gastrojejunostomy has been shown to provide some relief as it is able to provide gastric decompression, but it fails to completely address duodenal obstruction. By failing to relieve this obstruction, obstructive symptoms persist later requiring this be addressed, likely with a duodenojejunostomy. There is also the risk of blind loop syndrome, gastric bile reflux, and peptic ulceration as a result of the remaining obstruction [6, 17].

The Strong procedure involves the division of the ligament of Treitz allowing for caudal duodenal mobilization outside the aortomesenteric angle. The Strong procedure has been favored in the past as it is the least invasive procedure and maintains the bowel intact as it does not require anastomosis. However, it has been quoted to have a failure rate of at least 25%, which likely results from tethering of the inferior pancreaticoduodenal artery [5, 11, 17]. This failure rate is also likely due to the fact that it does not directly address the region of obstruction. Notably, Ganss et al. reported the case of a patient having undergone the strong procedure twice without symptomatic improvement each time. This further highlights the ineffectiveness of this procedure in treating SMAS. Our experience has similarly shown a low success rate relative to other surgical options.

Duodenojejunostomy has been the most accepted surgical treatment option. This is largely because it has yielded the most favorable results as compared to gastrojejunostomy and the Strong procedure. DDJ, open or laparoscopic, involves performing a side-to-side anastomosis involving the proximal jejunum and duodenum. Kroh et al. published outcomes on 18 patients who underwent DDJ and although 14 of 18 patients reported initial symptom improvement, only six patients reported intermediate symptomatic improvement or resolution. While uncommon, recurrence of symptoms has been described after duodenojejunostomy alone after the migration of the anastomosis under the SMA, thus recreating the previous obstruction [4, 20]. Performing a complete duodenal derotation mitigates this risk.

Duodenojejunostomy without the division of the fourth portion of the duodenum poses a risk of blind loop syndrome. To avoid this, a Roux-en-Y duodenojejunal bypass is a reasonable alternative as it leaves minimal possibility for blind loop syndrome [1, 6] (Fig. 8.4). This operation has been quoted to have a 90% success rate in the literature with improvement early in the postoperative period, though data is limited due to a lack of long-term follow-up [2, 3]. However, a series published by Chang et al. reports a 33% improvement or resolution of symptoms. Patients that experienced recurrence or persisting symptoms underwent full diagnostic workup, including imaging studies confirming patency of the anastomosis, concluding that recurrence or lack of significant improvement may be due to other chronic pain syndromes or gastrointestinal dysmotility syndromes. In this series, 2 out of 18 patients also developed a prolonged ileus postoperatively, which is

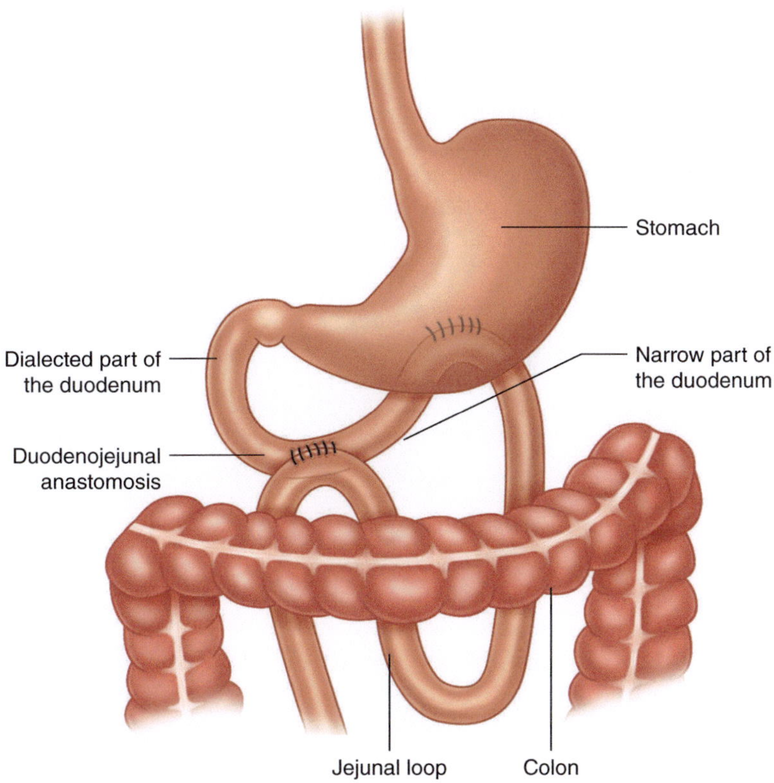

Fig. 8.4 Loop duodenojejunal bypass

consistent with the experience in our practice. It has not been our experience that a majority of patients experience significant improvement early in the postoperative period.

While the best treatment for SMAS remains unclear, in our practice and experience, duodenal derotation as described in the literature by Dr. Domingo Alvear, along with a duodenoduodenostomy, has been most effective in treating patients with SMAS. Alvear reported a series of 19 patients who underwent duodenal derotation, of which 18 had long-term symptomatic improvement or resolution. Seven of 19 patients required a second operation for persistent symptoms which improved with duodenoduodenostomy, however, it is important to note this is not explicitly mentioned in the manuscript. Two of the 18 patients required lysis of adhesions secondary to small bowel obstruction [8].

In our practice, the full condition of SMAS is addressed by performing a duodenal derotation, as described in the literature by Ha, Alvear, and Leber, with concurrent duodenoduodenostomy [8] (Fig. 8.5). In our experience, most patients develop a prolonged postoperative ileus and often experience delayed symptomatic improvement. It is our practice to routinely place a gastrojejunostomy tube at the time of, or prior to, surgery to allow for decompression of the stomach, providing the patient with relief and mitigating the risk of frequent bilious emesis postoperatively. The jejunal tube is placed past the area of anastomosis, when possible, to have a means of nutrition postoperatively. Furthermore, all patients go home with a PICC for IV hydration in the case of high gastric output and/or for parenteral nutrition for those who would otherwise struggle with enteral nutrition.

Lastly, it is important to note that psychiatric illness and other preexisting medical conditions may confuse a patient's clinical picture and should be taken into consideration with regard to patient selection [6]. There is a suggestion that

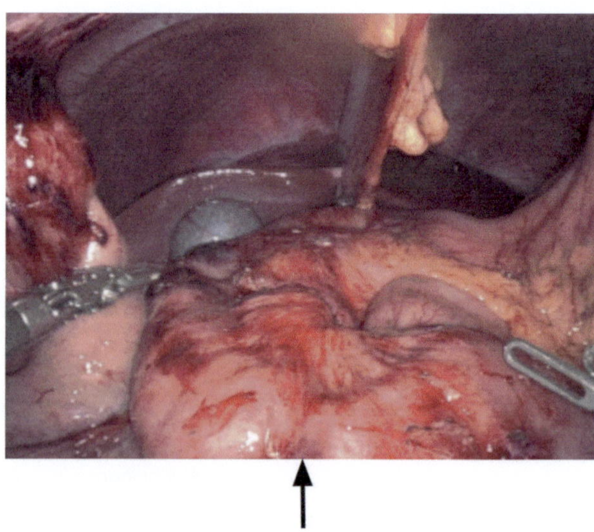

Fig. 8.5 After duodenal derotation with duodenum to the right of midline

preexisting psychiatric conditions, and, in our experience, signs and symptoms of intestinal dysmotility may be associated with prolonged persistence of symptoms and may be linked to lack of complete symptom resolution. It has also been our experience that patients unable to tolerate nasojejunal or gastrojejunal tube feeds at the goal rate are much less likely to experience significant improvement in pain and symptoms. Surgical intervention for SMAS serves the primary function of relieving a mechanical obstruction and does not address functional disorders, such as global intestinal dysmotility. Psychological management and intervention are also strongly recommended in the literature to ensure the best possible long-term outcomes in patients afflicted by psychiatric disorders. Literature has also indicated that very few of these patients are likely to benefit from surgical intervention, further emphasizing the importance of adequate patient selection [10]. It has also been suggested that this may be a poor outcome predictor for patients electing to undergo duodenojejunostomy for SMAS [6].

Conclusion

SMAS is a complex disease characterized by duodenal outlet obstruction secondary to compression of the third portion of the duodenum between the aorta and SMA. Up to 31% of patients diagnosed with SMAS develop it secondary to weight loss from MALS. Although many patients who develop SMAS do so because of rapid or profound weight loss, other etiologies have been described. SMAS is best diagnosed by measuring the aortomesenteric angle and distance with CT or MRI. An angle <18° and a distance <8 mm are highly specific for a diagnosis of SMAS in the right clinical context. If medical management is unsuccessful, several surgical options have been described, including gastrojejunostomy, duodenojejunostomy, and Strong procedure. In our experience, duodenal derotation with duodenoduodenostomy described by Domingo Alvear provides the highest possibility of success in relieving symptoms.

References

1. Merrett ND, Wilson RB, Cosman P, Biankin AV. Superior mesenteric artery syndrome: diagnosis and treatment strategies. J Gastrointest Surg. 2009;13(2):287–92. https://doi.org/10.1007/s11605-008-0695-4.
2. Chang J, Boules M, Rodriguez J, Walsh M, Rosenthal R, Kroh M. Laparoscopic duodenojejunostomy for superior mesenteric artery syndrome: intermediate follow-up results and a review of the literature. Surg Endosc. 2017;31(3):1180–5. https://doi.org/10.1007/s00464-016-5088-2.
3. Mandarry M, Zhao L, Zhang C, et al. A comprehensive review of superior mesenteric artery syndrome. Eur Surg. 2010;42:229–36. https://doi.org/10.1007/s10353-010-0561-y.
4. Fraser JD, Peter SD, Hughes JH, Swain JM. Laparoscopic duodenojejunostomy for superior mesenteric artery syndrome. JSLS. 2009;13(2):254–9.

5. Ganss A, Rampado S, Savarino E, Bardini R. Superior mesenteric artery syndrome: a prospective study in a single institution. J Gastrointest Surg. 2019;23(5):997–1005. https://doi.org/10.1007/s11605-018-3984-6.
6. Sun Z, Rodriguez J, McMichael J, et al. Minimally invasive duodenojejunostomy for superior mesenteric artery syndrome: a case series and review of the literature. Surg Endosc. 2015;29(5):1137–44. https://doi.org/10.1007/s00464-014-3775-4.
7. Biank V, Werlin S. Superior mesenteric artery syndrome in children: a 20-year experience. J Pediatr Gastroenterol Nutr. 2006;42(5):522–5. https://doi.org/10.1097/01.mpg.0000221888.36501.f2.
8. Ha CD, Alvear DT, Leber DC. Duodenal derotation as an effective treatment of superior mesenteric artery syndrome: a thirty-three year experience. Am Surg. 2008;74(7):644–53.
9. Van Horne N, Jackson JP. Superior mesenteric artery syndrome. In: StatPearls. Treasure Island: StatPearls Publishing; 2024. https://www-ncbi-nlm-nih-gov.mlprox.csmc.edu/books/NBK482209/.
10. Jonas JP, Rössler F, Ghafoor S, et al. Surgical therapy of celiac axis and superior mesenteric artery syndrome. Langenbeck's Arch Surg. 2023;408(1):59. https://doi.org/10.1007/s00423-023-02803-w.
11. Pottorf BJ, Husain FA, Hollis HW, Lin E. Laparoscopic management of duodenal obstruction resulting from superior mesenteric artery syndrome. JAMA Surg. 2014;149(12):1319–22. https://doi.org/10.1001/jamasurg.2014.1409.
12. Ozkurt H, Cenker MM, Bas N, Erturk SM, Basak M. Measurement of the distance and angle between the aorta and superior mesenteric artery: normal values in different BMI categories. Surg Radiol Anat. 2007;29(7):595–9. https://doi.org/10.1007/s00276-007-0238-9.
13. Sapkas G, O'Brien JP. Vascular compression of the duodenum (cast syndrome) associated with the treatment of spinal deformities. A report of six cases. Arch Orthop Trauma Surg. 1981;98(1):7–11. https://doi.org/10.1007/BF00389703.
14. Akin JT Jr, Gray SW, Skandalakis JE. Vascular compression of the duodenum: presentation of ten cases and review of the literature. Surgery. 1976;79(5):515–22.
15. Strong EK. Mechanics of arteriomesenteric duodenal obstruction and direct surgical attack upon etiology. Ann Surg. 1958;148(5):725–30. https://doi.org/10.1097/00000658-195811000-00001.
16. Record J, Morris B, Adolph V. Resolution of refractory superior mesenteric artery syndrome with laparoscopic duodenojejunostomy: pediatric case series with spectrum of clinical imaging. Ochsner J. 2015;15(1):74–8. https://www.ncbi.nlm.nih.gov/pmc/articles/PMC4365851/.
17. Welsch T, Büchler MW, Kienle P. Recalling superior mesenteric artery syndrome. Dig Surg. 2007;24(3):149–56. https://doi.org/10.1159/000102097.
18. Nguyen LA, Snape WJ. Clinical presentation and pathophysiology of gastroparesis. Gastroenterol Clin N Am. 2015;44(1):21–30. https://doi.org/10.1016/j.gtc.2014.11.003.
19. Unal B, Aktaş A, Kemal G, et al. Superior mesenteric artery syndrome: CT and ultrasonography findings. Diagn Interv Radiol. 2005;11(2):90–5.
20. Raissi B, Taylor BM, Taves DH. Recurrent superior mesenteric artery (Wilkie's) syndrome: a case report. Can J Surg. 1996;39(5):410–6.

Chapter 9
Nonoperative Management of Median Arcuate Ligament Syndrome

Benjamin Abraham and Clement Ho

Introduction

According to some estimates, healthcare spending in the United States is projected to double over the next 10 years, without an accompanying increase in healthcare outcomes across the board. Survival after myocardial infarction is similar in both the United States and Canada, but expenditures in the United States were between 5 and 10 times greater to achieve the same outcome [1].

Multiple studies have affirmed the value of preoperative optimization of the surgical patient to improve postoperative results [2]. In the case of median arcuate ligament syndrome (MALS), the disease often travels together with a variety of other complex comorbid conditions including:

- Malnutrition.
- Inheritable connective tissue disorders.
- Depression/anxiety.
- Postural orthostatic tachycardia syndrome (POTS).
- Fibromyalgia.
- Other abdominal vascular abnormalities.

Therefore, our approach at the initial consult has been to actively screen for comorbid conditions and optimize the health of the whole patient, in preparation for the potential of general anesthesia and surgery.

Initial presentation can vary greatly, including the patient-reported location of pain (epigastric, periumbilical, sternal, costal, thoracolumbar, or flank) and timing (episodic, continuous, postprandial, exercise-induced, postoperative) [3]. Furthermore, preoperative symptoms often vary from postoperative pain when there

B. Abraham (✉) · C. Ho
Department of Anesthesiology and Pain Management, Cleveland Clinic, Cleveland, OH, USA
e-mail: abrahab@ccf.org

D. Shouhed et al. (eds.), *Median Arcuate Ligament Syndrome*,
https://doi.org/10.1007/978-3-031-80740-4_9

are residual or refractory symptoms. A long roster of varied subspecialists is commonplace for many patients, even prior to presenting to our clinic. Here, we see a great opportunity to begin the conversation on an algorithmic approach to MALS for the proper selection and perioperative optimization of the patient, in order to maximize postoperative outcome.

As the surgical treatment for MALS has evolved over time, so too has our approach. Emerging research, including imaging of asymptomatic family members, seems to suggest an underlying genetic basis for the disease, though incompletely characterized and poorly understood at this time [4, 5]. Other authors have posited that the pain of MALS is chiefly neuropathic rather than vascular in origin [6], with important similarities to traumatic neuroma [7, 8]. We concur with this conclusion, and our approach at initial consultation has evolved over the last decade. We've used lessons learned from our multicenter, multidisciplinary collaboration to focus on the evidence-based tools to treat this neuropathic pain syndrome.

Patient Education

Prior to any medical or surgical intervention, it is essential for the patient to identify their goal or endpoint for treatment, discuss this with the interdisciplinary treatment team, and have it documented in the medical record [9]. This may be a very foreign idea to the patient and family; the end goal of heart valve replacement would be replacement of a faulty valve, restoration of normal flow across the valve, and return of balance to the cardiac cycle. Meanwhile, the patient's goal of this very same surgery may be to "walk the dog" or "mow the lawn." Neither the lawn nor the dog walking is *objectively* measured at the first postoperative visit, *though it may be the top-most priority of the patient.* We therefore underscore the concept of "functional restoration" with the patient and family at the initial consultation, along with the need for an objective means to measure it.

There is strong evidence that the numeric rating scale (NRS), erroneously labeled "the fifth vital sign" is not an adequate outcome measure for success [10], especially when applied to abdominal pain syndromes. Our patients have typically valued weight gain (or the stemming of ongoing weight loss), return to work/school, and caloric/macro- and micronutrient intake reflected by laboratory testing. In other painful syndromes, "pain reduction" was a highly ranked goal, but not without a concomitant increase in physical function measures. We have learned a great deal from the treatment of other abdominal pain syndromes, in particular inflammatory bowel disease and endometriosis. Without goal identification and documentation pretreatment, there is the risk that the "endpoint" of treatment will shift, ever-advancing just out of reach of the patient-physician team, just over the horizon. This frustration is often shared by everyone involved in the care of this often complex condition. Precisely defining a relevant treatment goal prior to surgery is critical for successful recovery postoperatively [9].

Non-Pharmacologic Treatment

For a wide variety of painful conditions, exercise therapy has been shown to improve patient-reported numerical pain scores. This phenomenon, called exercise-induced hypoalgesia (EIH), has been shown to reduce pain perception to noxious stimuli and appears to last at least 30 min postexercise. Much of the available literature on painful conditions focuses on the perception of pain and patient report of impact on their life. Aerobic, anaerobic, and resistance exercises all appear to activate EIH in healthy volunteers. However, the incidence of increased pain sensitivity after exercise is prominent in chronic pain populations, and experimental studies suggest chronic pain patients show significant impairment of the EIH response [11]. Histologic data corroborates the role of the N-methyl D- aspartate (NMDA) receptor within the pain signaling pathways, playing a key role in pain sensitization and modulation [12, 13].

Various studies have suggested higher body mass index correlates well with lower celiac peak systolic velocity, as well as wider celiac artery diameter. While poorly understood, it is believed that the greater degree of adipose tissue surrounding the median arcuate ligament decreases the susceptibility of the celiac artery and celiac plexus to compression [14]. We would also acknowledge that in pediatric patients, changes in height also appear to change the degree to which compression of the celiac axis occurs. Analogously, we concur with reports suggesting that changes to the Cobb angle following scoliosis surgery can lead to worsening (or improvement) of symptoms based on changes in celiac axis geometry. Therefore, we were not surprised to see that manipulation of the local nerve-artery relationship may be possible with certain physical maneuvers.

Yoga

For centuries, yoga has been used as an adjuvant treatment for both common and rare painful conditions. Studies evaluating the efficacy of yoga for the treatment of chronic back pain, for example, have shown modest improvement in symptom reports as well as objective physical measurements. There, yoga has been shown to be noninferior to traditional physical therapy [15–17]. It has long been hypothesized that *agnisara* stimulates the parasympathetic system to stimulate “digestion” [18]. For MALS, manipulation of the diaphragmatic position in relation to the celiac axis appears to change the degree of compression or at least the symptoms of compression. Reports of agnisara yoga impacting “digestion” and “digestive health” have been around since medieval times. Modern investigations have borne out this ancient belief; Minvaleev et al. demonstrated an increase in superior mesenteric artery diameter, along with increases in SMA blood flow confirmed by ultrasound, as a direct result of yogic movements in the novice. In theory, the *upward-facing dog and* a*gnisara* mimic deep inspiration. Repeated retraction of the abdominal muscles appears to provide benefits when done on a regular basis [19]. In our own practice, we routinely recommend upward-facing dog (urdhva mukha svanasana), andagnisara with uddiyana bandha, and would agree with other authors that a modest improvement in symptoms can be achieved in motivated MALS patients. A mean increase of 6.6% in arterial diameter accompanied by 12.7% mean increase in SMA blood flow also appears to correlate well with our clinical experience for the celiac axis; a small but meaningful benefit is attained in those able to adhere to the yogic regimen. This is especially relevant in the physically deconditioned patient preparing for the stress of general anesthesia and surgery.

Physical Therapy

For a variety of painful conditions, we have used preoperative physical therapy as an adjunct to treatment, in anticipation of the early mobilization required for effective postoperative recovery. We have seen small improvements in MALS symptoms with physical therapy. Muscle strengthening, lordosis reduction, and diaphragm mobilization appear to work similarly to yoga by strengthening the rectus abdominis, transverse abdominus, pelvic floor, lower trapezius, rhomboids, and latissimus dorsi. Positions favoring reduction of lumbar lordosis have been strongly associated with reduced MALS-related pain [20]. In our team-based approach, we use a combination of physical therapy, yoga, and cognitive behavior therapy. This approach takes advantage of the aforementioned exercise-induced hypoalgesia (EIH) [21] and simultaneously addresses comorbid psychological/psychiatric diseases, which frequently can inhibit postsurgical recovery.

Medication Optimization

The use of prescription opioids in the treatment of low back pain is extremely common, despite limited evidence of long-term benefit. Evidence suggests worsened surgical outcomes following spine surgery, correlating well with increasing morphine equivalents (MEDs). Among adults presenting for initial MALS evaluation in our clinic, approximately 70% are currently taking chronic opioid medications as an outpatient. We have also found a higher-than-anticipated percentage of pediatric patients treated with chronic opioid therapy, especially when compared to non-MALS pediatric patients. Not surprisingly, chronic opioid therapy for non-cancer, nonsurgical abdominal pain has failed to improve outcomes when compared to its non-opioid counterparts. In recent years, the use of chronic opioid therapy for non-cancer pain has fallen out of favor due to abuse, systemic side effects, and opioid-induced hyperalgesia (OIH) [22]. In the context of MALS and general anesthesia, opioid tolerance preoperatively has been associated with increased requirements intra- and postoperatively. Furthermore, the use of intravenous opioids during general anesthesia appears to have far-reaching consequences during recovery. This has led to a number of centers, including ours, to taper the patients preoperatively and/or avoid opioid therapy entirely during certain types of general anesthesia [23]. Instead, we rely on regional anesthesia and non-opioid adjuvant medications where possible [24]. There have been a variety of setbacks in this effort, including a large body of fraudulent research intermingled with well-conducted trials on multimodal analgesia [25].

Pharmacologic Management of MALS-Related Symptoms

There is currently no standardized approach for the nonsurgical treatment of median arcuate ligament syndrome. There exists a large armamentarium of highly effective analgesics available for other chronic pain conditions. We have tailored our approach to include lessons learned from other neuropathic pain conditions, as well as other causes of chronic abdominal pain.

Ketamine

Ketamine is a commonly used anesthetic and analgesic, acting as both an opioid receptor agonist and NMDA receptor antagonist. Ketamine's bronchodilatory properties, along with maintenance of spontaneous breathing, make it a highly useful medication. The NMDA receptor is an excitatory glutaminergic receptor, found in both spinal and supraspinal sites, and is responsible for afferent nociceptive signal transmission. In chronic pain states, these receptors appear to be upregulated, resulting in amplified pain signals via central sensitization. Outside of the operating room, the action of ketamine on NMDA receptor antagonism has proven highly effective for the treatment of refractory neuropathic pain.

Meta-analyses have demonstrated the usefulness of this medication for phantom limb pain, neuropathic cancer pain, complex regional pain syndrome, fibromyalgia, and ischemic limb pain. Oral ketamine has not seen similar widespread usage, most likely due to limitations by first-pass metabolism. In contrast to IV ketamine, evidence for the use of oral ketamine is lacking, with most studies being underpowered with a small sample size [26]. Intranasal ketamine has high bioavailability [27] and is frequently used in well-selected patients as a 5% or 10% solution [28]. In our practice, we have found compounded intranasal preparations of ketamine to be especially effective in those patients with residual or recurrent MALS symptoms who are unable to unwilling to undergo reoperation. Compared to intravenous preparations administered in a hospital setting, outpatient treatment with intranasal ketamine has proven to be more easily accessible to the patient, as well as cost-effective from an insurance coverage perspective.

Esketamine, a ketamine enantiomer, is an FDA-approved medication for treatment-refractory major depression but lacks labeling for other neuropathic conditions. Anecdotally, we have found reports of symptomatic improvement, including improvement on patient-reported quality-of-life survey measures, in those incidentally treated with this agent for depression. Recruitment for the adequately powered study of those patients using esketamine for treatment-refractory major depression and who also have symptomatic MALS anatomy has been challenging. Further randomized study on this topic is needed [29]. There are no commercially available ketamine solutions labeled for outpatient administration, but compounding by both inpatient and outpatient pharmacies is readily available.

While numerous protocols exist, we have settled on a 4-h infusion regimen of intravenous ketamine in the outpatient setting. For refractory neuropathic pain, including for MALS symptoms refractory to surgical treatment, we titrate to a goal of 0.5 mg/kg/h if tolerated. Close monitoring is required due to possible (albeit rare) psychomimetic, gastrointestinal, and cardiac effects. To that end, we exclude patients with poorly controlled angina, elevated intracranial pressure, history of psychosis, and severe liver/renal disease [30, 31].

Tricyclic Antidepressants (TCAs)

The tricyclic antidepressant group of medications are serotonin and noradrenaline reuptake inhibitors with additional antagonist effects on alpha-1, alpha-2 adrenergic, and H1 histamine receptors. Currently, amitriptyline, imipramine, nortriptyline, and desipramine are most commonly prescribed to treat neuropathic pain, though they each have slightly different mechanistic effects.

The NMDA receptor and ion channel (sodium and calcium) blocking properties are proposed to augment the TCA effect on pain modulation [32]. Structures such as the anterior cingulate cortex, prefrontal cortex, thalamus, hippocampus, insular cortex, and amygdala are involved in both pain and mood. Perception of pain, particularly of chronic abdominal pain, could therefore be thought of as "the memory of pain" that persists. Histologic evidence suggests long-term changes in neuronal connectivity in the brain and spinal cord [33]. Hence, the synergism between chronic abdominal pain and various mood disorders (e.g., depression) can act to worsen the symptoms of both. This synergy, and the widespread overlap in treatment, is particularly relevant in our experience with MALS.

Increasing evidence suggests a wide variety of disorders co-occur with MALS including fibromyalgia. This parallels our own clinical experience. In our practice, tricyclic antidepressants such as amitriptyline are commonly used as first-line treatments for neuropathic "central pain syndromes" such as fibromyalgia. At the initial consult preoperatively, we offer low-dose tricyclic antidepressant-type medications as a first-line medication for MALS. According to a Cochrane Library Review, encompassing 15 studies, the use of amitriptyline dosing from 25 mg to 200 mg per day only benefits well-selected patients for specific conditions and is not the abdominal pain panacea we once believed it to be [34]. In particular, amitriptyline has been shown to provide significant improvement of symptoms in pediatric functional abdominal pain (FAPD), with similar results to SSRIs. At 12 weeks, amitriptyline 10 mg (for children less than 35 kg, or 25 mg for children weighing over 35 kg) has shown quality of life improvements, as well as reduction in subjective pain report without major side effect [35].

Nortriptyline, the primary active metabolite of amitriptyline, is not licensed to treat neuropathic pain in the USA but is recommended around the world. Doses of 10–75 mg once daily are recommended. However, according to Cochrane Library systematic review, there is insufficient evidence for nortriptyline's efficacy in neuropathic pain conditions. Nortriptyline remains a part of our treatment plan for those that do not tolerate other medications, due to its low cost and benign side effect profile [36].

Anticonvulsants

Anti-epilepsy drugs (AEDs), also known as anticonvulsants, are a diverse group of medications frequently used in our practice as first-line agents in the pre- and post-surgical patient with neuropathic pain. The pain-relieving effects occur through a variety of different mechanisms. Benzodiazepines and barbiturates are GABA-A receptor agonists. Phenytoin, carbamazepine, and valproate are sodium channel blockers. Due to the monitoring requirements, side effect profile, and potential for abuse, none of these agents are used in our clinic.

In contrast, so-called gabapentinoids such as pregabalin and gabapentin are widely prescribed in our practice as first-line agents. These medications act on the calcium channel rather than via GABA itself. The alpha 2-delta-1 (A2d-1) isoform of voltage-gated calcium channel is responsible for pain signal transmission and is mostly found in the cerebral cortex, hippocampus, and cerebellum in animal models.

Gabapentinoids appear to exert their effect by binding to alpha 2-delta-1 subunit and modulate the presynaptic excitatory input onto dorsal horn ganglion [37]. A2d-1 is essential for nerve injury-induced pre- and postsynaptic NMDA receptor hyperactivity, and we believe this pathway is of great importance in the pathophysiology of MALS [38].

Gabapentinoids also appear to exert a poorly understood effect on neuroinflammation in the central nervous system [39], whose effect is responsible for a variety of central nervous system mediated pain conditions including fibromyalgia. Systematic reviews of gabapentin have demonstrated wide applicability for these medications in a variety of chronic neuropathic pain syndromes. Gabapentin doses of 1800–3600 mg/day, in divided doses, provide significant pain reduction for patients with postherpetic neuralgia and diabetic peripheral neuropathy. However, there is limited evidence on the dose-response effect for patients with other chronic neuropathic pain. Not surprisingly, gabapentin and its derivatives remain the mainstay of treatment in our clinic for MALS [40], though further study is needed. Another meta-analysis on the effectiveness of gabapentin and pregabalin on sciatic-type neuropathic pain shows significant relief in radicular leg pain at 2 weeks, and again further improvement at 3 months. However, pregabalin and gabapentin did not provide better pain relief and functionality after 52 weeks and 8 weeks compared to placebo, respectively. We would agree with that time course in regard to

MALS; it is well suited for the patient contemplating MAL surgery but not yet scheduled.

While it is important to note the possible adverse effects associated with pregabalin and gabapentin (e.g., drowsiness, dizziness, nausea [41]), we have not found this to be a significant dose-limiting factor in MALS. Perhaps because of the relatively young age of our MALS patient population, these medications have been well-tolerated in therapeutic doses. Discontinuation due to these dose-limiting side effects accounts for less than 1% of cases in our practice. In contrast, where we have found failures with a single agent, it is due to incomplete analgesia at our ceiling of 900 mg four times daily. Therefore, we instead encourage a multifaceted attack on the symptoms as described below, using multiple treatment modalities simultaneously.

With surgical treatment being the end goal, our plan for MALS usually involves instructions to taper the medication in the postoperative period, in the weeks or months after operation. Labeled elsewhere for the treatment of anxiety, gabapentinoids continued long-term may be exerting action on other benefits for comorbid psychiatric conditions. Our experience has been that a significant proportion of patients will self-discontinue gabapentinoids in the postoperative period, with assistance from local pediatricians or internists, and are frequently lost to follow up with us thereafter.

Carbamazepine and oxcarbazepine are considered first-line therapies for trigeminal neuralgia (TN). Carbamazepine 800–1200 mg/day and oxcarbazepine 600–1800 mg/day provide significant initial pain control in 90% of trigeminal neuralgia patients [42]. In the MALS patient, however, our experience has shown these medications to be poorly tolerated due to monitoring requirements as well as somnolence at therapeutic doses. Topiramate is another commonly used treatment for chronic neuropathic pain. However, in a Cochrane review in 2016, topiramate dosing of 100 mg and up to 400 mg daily provided no benefit in those suffering from diabetic neuropathy or fibromyalgia. We would caution that the use of this medication be restricted to only well-selected MALS patients who have a significant component of migraine headache, with careful monitoring for the weight loss often associated with this treatment [43].

Selective Serotonin Reuptake Inhibitors (SSRI)

Selective serotonin reuptake inhibitors (SSRI) are a non-tricyclic family of drugs that increase the binding time at the serotonin receptor by inhibiting the reuptake of serotonin. This class includes citalopram, escitalopram, fluoxetine, paroxetine, and sertraline. SSRIs lack the norepinephrine reuptake inhibition and postsynaptic and ion channel blockade seen with TCAs. Functional abdominal pain in pediatric patients as well as irritable bowel syndrome are often treated with SSRIs, where cognitive behavioral therapy and other non-pharmacologic treatments have failed.

In adults and children, chronic abdominal pain is associated with visceral hyperalgesia (sometimes called visceral hypersensitivity). It is a pathological state where the threshold for pain sensation in response to gastrointestinal sensory stimulus is lowered, often dramatically. We suspect that there may be a connection between MALS and the increased sensitivity to noxious and non-noxious stimuli.

The mechanism of analgesia for SSRIs) in functional abdominal pain is believed to be via modulation of visceral hypersensitivity, in addition to increasing digestive tract transit time and augmenting the analgesic effect of other agents. The strong association between chronic abdominal pain and psychological symptoms, such as anxiety and depression, makes antidepressant use more favorable for many of our patients. Studies comparing the efficacy of SSRI vs. TCA in pediatric chronic abdominal pain suggest better outcomes with SSRI on patient-reported pain scales, accompanied by less severe side effects, even after correcting for psychological comorbidities and other interventions. This is in contrast with the superior therapeutic effect of TCAs for adults when compared to SSRI agents in the treatment of peripheral neuropathy and chronic abdominal pain [44]. According to a recent review, there are multiple studies performed on the use of citalopram on functional abdominal pain. Citalopram doses from 10 to 40 mg/day show a therapeutic effect independent of patient's psychological baseline [45].

We frequently encounter patients with a prior diagnosis of fibromyalgia. Often, they carry this diagnosis as an alternative explanation for gastrointestinal symptoms of MALS. Fibromyalgia appears to be caused by dysfunction of pain processing at the central nervous system level rather than a discrete musculoskeletal injury in the periphery [46]. SSRIs are commonly used in the treatment of fibromyalgia and appear to mitigate the effects of both pain and comorbid psychological disease. Some evidence exists for the use of SSRIs, such as citalopram, fluoxetine, and paroxetine, providing a 30% reduction in numerical pain scores compared to placebo. There remains a debate on the benefits of SSRI) use for the reduction of secondary outcomes such as fatigue, anxiety, physical debility, as well as quality of life and sleep quality. Sertraline and citalopram, though commonly used in chronic pelvic pain, have not been widely beneficial in our treatment of MALS-related pain. Similarly, fluoxetine has been shown to provide significant pain reduction in fibromyalgia, migraine, chronic pelvic pain, and diabetic peripheral neuropathy, though it has been met with little success in our practice with MALS. Paroxetine appears to improve patient-reported quality of life measures, improvements in anxiety and depression, without reducing pain scores [47].

Serotonin Norepinephrine Reuptake Inhibitors (SNRI)

Serotonin norepinephrine reuptake inhibitors (SNRI) are a family of drugs that increase both serotonin and noradrenaline receptors binding time and intensity by inhibiting the reuptake of both neurotransmitters. This drug class includes duloxetine, venlafaxine, and desvenlafaxine. SNRIs, like SSRIs, exert their pain modulation effect by directly decreasing neuronal activity along the nociceptive pathway, both in the CNS and PNS [48]. Venlafaxine, one of the first SNRIs to be approved by the FDA for treatment of psychiatric disorders such as panic disorder, social phobia, and major depression, has long been used off-label for neuropathic pain, with effective dosing at 150 mg/day or higher.

Duloxetine is recommended by the European Federation of Neurological Societies (EFNS), Neuropathic Pain Special Interest Group (NeuPSIG), and National Institute for Health and Care Excellence (NICE) as a first-line treatment for neuropathic pain. Despite its widespread use in diabetic- and chemotherapy-induced peripheral neuropathy [49, 50], we have found that dose-dependent exacerbations of insomnia and nausea [51] have limited its usefulness in patients with MALS.

Magnesium

Magnesium sulfate has been used for both acute and chronic pain conditions. The main mechanism of action appears to be via an antagonist effect on N-methyl-D-aspartate receptors. NMDA receptors, when activated by glutamate, allow for the influx of calcium ions. By inhibiting calcium influx, magnesium can decrease central sensitization and attenuate pain hypersensitivity [52]. Intravenous (IV) magnesium sulfate provides significant pain reduction in patients with abdominal pain, peripheral neuropathy, complex regional pain syndrome, fibromyalgia, and lower back pain. The recommended IV magnesium dose is 30–50 mg/kg bolus with 6–20 mg/kg/h continuous infusion [53]. Oral magnesium formulations (magnesium malate, magnesium oxide, magnesium pidolate, or magnesium citrate) also showed modest analgesic effect in outpatient settings according to several randomized, double-blind, placebo-controlled, crossover studies. The dosing for oral magnesium used in these studies ranges from 9 mg/kg to 4500 mg daily [54]. We have been surprised to find that prior to our initial consult visit for MALS, many patients have already begun titrating oral magnesium via over-the-counter preparations.

Diagnostic Nerve Blockade

In our own practice, we have found great variation in symptomatology on initial presentation. For this reason, the disease is often difficult to diagnose in the primary care setting, and difficult to effectively treat without the assistance of multiple subspecialists. Treatment success depends heavily on careful patient selection and avoidance of confounding factors. When there is a high pretest probability for a diagnosis of MALS (e.g., concordant symptoms, physical exam, and imaging) our protocol is to perform diagnostic nerve blockade to help predict the postsurgical outcome of MAL release. Importantly, response to diagnostic celiac plexus blockade does not appear to correlate with the presence of arterial abnormalities alone. As such, we no longer use celiac artery patency as a standalone exclusion criterion for MALS [5].

Where possible, we have used the percutaneous transaortic approach to the celiac plexus in order to more precisely target the region of surgical interest. We use fluoroscopic or computed tomography for image guidance. In cases of thoracolumbar spinal hardware or deformity, we have collaborated with gastroenterology for an endoscopic ultrasound-guided approach instead. Though its inclusion is common at other institutions, for all diagnostic blockades, we omit corticosteroids entirely and instead choose a very low volume of long-acting local anesthetic (e.g., ropivacaine).

The choice of procedural sedation or anesthesia appears to impact the sensitivity of diagnostic blockade. Subhypnotic doses of propofol have long been suspected to exert a direct anti-emetic effect. Depending on the propofol dose and type of surgery, this effect appears to vary from none at all to 30 minutes to 24 hours [55, 56]. While recent well-conducted studies from our own institution have cast some doubt on this effect [57], it remains a confounding factor in our choice of anesthetic for diagnostic blockade in MALS. We avoid it where possible and find pre-procedure patient education to be a useful and effective substitute for general anesthesia in this minimally invasive percutaneous procedure.

Low doses of midazolam are commonly used for moderate sedation during diagnostic celiac plexus blockade. Again, there is a concern for a direct anti-nausea effect with benzodiazepines [58] causing interference with the accuracy of diagnostic blockade. Conversely, the use of pain-relieving agents during procedural sedation or anesthesia (e.g., fentanyl) is often strongly emetogenic. We strictly limit the use of intravenous opioid agonists during the procedure for this reason. Less than 10% of our patients opt for a local anesthetic only approach, forgoing anesthesia altogether.

Other Methods of Diagnostic and Therapeutic Nerve Blockade

Where prior stenting, prior surgery, or arterial calcification limits the transaortic approach to the celiac plexus, we use a splanchnic nerve blockade for diagnostic purposes instead.

Though previously used in many centers (including our own), differential epidural blockade for diagnostic purposes has fallen out of favor for the diagnosis of visceral pain syndromes. It is both time-intensive and vulnerable to multiple confounding factors in this situation [59] with a low sensitivity and specificity.

Abdominal cutaneous nerve entrapment syndrome (ACNES) can contribute to pain in patients with multiple prior abdominal surgeries and extensive scar tissue. Where no vascular surgery is pending, we use a therapeutic ultrasound-guided transverse abdominis plane (TAP) blockade with botulinum toxin rather than local anesthetic only.

As with other causes of chronic abdominal pain (e.g., chronic pancreatitis), we have had limited success with the use of celiac plexus neurolysis, spinal cord stimulation, and intrathecal drug delivery in treatment-refractory MALS. While anecdotal evidence exists, further investigation of these modalities is needed before incorporation into our treatment algorithm.

Summary

"Empirical research [suggests] that patients with severe illnesses prefer the physician to dominate [the] decision processes and provide the information needed. However, in rare diseases, due to the low prevalence and the lack of expertise, the patient is forced to become knowledgeable about his own disease state. Here, the patient often becomes an expert in his disease." [60].

In the case of MALS, these findings are particularly relevant. The patients are often young, technologically savvy, and exposed to an overwhelming amount of information on the disease, without definitive conclusions on its management. The problem arises when the patient (and parents) lack the tools to discern fact from fiction (or mere speculation) in the non-peer-reviewed literature. In truth, many of our patient referrals come from word-of-mouth and social media suggestions. In these domains, the presence of the physician and physician-scientist are almost entirely absent. While much work remains to be done on the topic, we offer this chapter as a starting point to discuss standardization in both the operative and nonoperative care of these challenging patients.

References

1. Mahajan A, Esper SA, Cole DJ, Fleisher LA. Anesthesiologists' role in value-based perioperative care and healthcare transformation. Anesthesiology. 2021;134:526–40.
2. Yerneni K, Nichols N, Abecassis ZA, Karras CL, Tan LA. Preoperative opioid use and clinical outcomes in spine surgery: a systematic review. Neurosurgery. 2020;86(6):E490–507.
3. Gloviczki P, Duncan AA. Treatment of celiac artery compression syndrome: does it really exist? Perspect Vasc Surg Endovasc Ther. 2007;19(3):259–63.
4. Okten RS, Kucukay F, Tola M, Bostanci B, Cumhur T. Is celiac artery compression syndrome genetically inherited?: a case series from a family and review of the literature. Eur J Radiol. 2012;81(6):1089–93.
5. Barbon DA, Hsu R, Noga J, Lazzara B, Miller T, Stainken BF. Clinical response to celiac plexus block confirms the neurogenic etiology of median arcuate ligament syndrome. J Vasc Interv Radiol. 2021;32(7):1081–7.
6. Weber JM, Boules M, Fong K, Abraham B, Bena J, El-Hayek K, Kroh M, Park WM. Median arcuate ligament syndrome is not a vascular disease. Ann Vasc Surg. 2016;30:22–7.
7. Chaum M, Shouhed D, Kim S, Walts AE, Marchevsky AM. Clinico-pathologic findings in patients with median arcuate ligament syndrome (celiac artery compression syndrome). Ann Diagn Pathol. 2021;52:151732.

8. Kwon JH, Ryu SW, Kang YN. Traumatic neuroma around the celiac trunk after gastrectomy mimicking a nodal metastasis: a case report. Korean J Radiol. 2007;8(3):242–5.
9. Goudman L, DeSmedt A, Linderoth B, Eldabe S, Witkam R, Henssen D, Moens M. Identifying goals in patients with chronic pain: a European survey. Eur J Pain. 2021;25(9):1090–3801.
10. Ballantyne J. Intensity of chronic pain—the wrong metric? N Engl J Med. 2015;373:2098–9.
11. Rice D, Nijs J, Kosek E, et al. Exercise-induced hypoalgesia in pain-free and chronic pain populations: state of the art and future directions. J Pain. 2019;20(11):1249–66.
12. Raja SN, Sivanesan E, Guan Y. Central sensitization, N-methyl-D-aspartate receptors, and human experimental pain models: bridging the gap between target discovery and drug development. Anesthesiology. 2019;131(2):233–5.
13. Liu YJ, Li YL, Fang ZH, Liao HL, Zhang YY, Lin J, Liu F, Shen JF. NMDARs mediate peripheral and central sensitization contributing to chronic orofacial pain. Front Cell Neurosci. 2022;16:999509.
14. Asbeutah AM, Bakir YY, Swamy N, Absuetah AAA, Abu-Asi MA, Sharma P. Subject body mass index affects Doppler waveform in celiac artery by duplex ultrasound. Open Cardiovasc Med J. 2013;7:40–5.
15. Zhu F, Zhang M, Wang D, Hong Q, Zeng C, Chen W. Yoga compared to non-exercise or physical therapy exercise on pain, disability, and quality of life for patients with chronic low back pain: a systematic review and meta-analysis of randomized controlled trials. PLoS One. 2020;15(9):e0238544.
16. Wieland LS, Skoetz N, Pilkington K, Vempati R, D'Adamo CR, Berman BM. Yoga treatment for chronic non-specific low back pain. Cochrane Database Syst Rev. 2017;1(1):CD010671.
17. Saper RB, Lemaster C, Delitto A, et al. Yoga, physical therapy, or education for chronic low Back pain: a randomized noninferiority trial. Ann Intern Med. 2017;167(2):85–94.
18. Minvaleev RS, Bogdanov RR, Kuznetsov AA, Bahner DP, Levitov AB. Yogic agnisara increases blood flow in the superior mesenteric artery. J Bodyw Mov Ther. 2022;31:97–101.
19. Ashish. Agnisar Kriya: meaning, steps, anatomy, benefits. FITSRI. Published December 23, 2020.
20. Janssen SL, Scholbach T, Jeno S, Laurie H, Meyer M, Combs C. Interprofessional management of median arcuate ligament syndrome (Dunbar syndrome) related to lumbar lordosis and hip dysplasia: a patient's perspective. Eur J Case Rep Intern Med. 2020;7(7):001605.
21. Archer KR, Devin CJ, Vanston SW, et al. Cognitive-behavioral-based physical therapy for patients with chronic pain undergoing lumbar spine surgery: a randomized controlled trial. J Pain. 2016;17(1):76–89.
22. Deyo RA, Von Korff M, Duhrkoop D. Opioids for low back pain. BMJ. 2015;350:g6380.
23. Coluzzi F, Bifulco F, Cuomo A, Dauri M, Leonardi C, Melotti RM, Natoli S, Romualdi P, Savoia G, Corcione A. The challenge of perioperative pain management in opioid-tolerant patients. Ther Clin Risk Manag. 2017;13:1163–73.
24. Siddiqui NT, Fischer H, Guerina L, Friedman Z. Effect of a preoperative gabapentin on post-operative analgesia in patients with inflammatory bowel disease following major bowel surgery: a randomized, placebo-controlled trial. Pain Pract. 2014;14(2):132–9.
25. McHugh UM, Yentis SM. An analysis of retractions of papers authored by Scott Reuben, Joachim Boldt and Yoshitaka Fujii. Anaesthesia. 2019;74(1):17–21. Erratum in: Anaesthesia. 2019;74(1):113
26. Blonk MI, Koder BG, van den Bemt PMLA, Huygen FJPM. Use of oral ketamine in chronic pain management: a review. Eur J Pain. 2010;14(5):466–72.
27. Yanagihara Y, Ohtani M, Kariya S, et al. Plasma concentration profiles of ketamine and norketamine after administration of various ketamine preparations to healthy Japanese volunteers. Biopharm Drug Dispos. 2003;24(1):37–43.
28. Carr DB, Goudas LC, Denman WT, et al. Safety and efficacy of intranasal ketamine for the treatment of breakthrough pain in patients with chronic pain: a randomized, double-blind, placebo-controlled, crossover study. Pain. 2004;108(1-2):17–27.

29. Fernandes M, Schelotto M, Doldi PM, et al. IMPORTANCE trial: a provisional study-design of a single-center, phase II, double-blinded, placebo-controlled, randomized, 4-week study to compare the efficacy and safety of intranasal esketamine in chronic opioid refractory pain. F1000Res. 2021;10:42.
30. Cohen SP, Bhatia A, Buvanendran A, et al. Consensus guidelines on the use of intravenous ketamine infusions for chronic pain from the American Society of Regional Anesthesia and Pain Medicine, the American Academy of Pain Medicine, and the American Society of Anesthesiologists. Reg Anesth Pain Med. 2018;43(5):521–46.
31. Niesters M, Martini C, Dahan A. Ketamine for chronic pain: risks and benefits. Br J Clin Pharmacol. 2014;77(2):357–67.
32. Sindrup SH, Otto M, Finnerup NB, Jensen TS. Antidepressants in the treatment of neuropathic pain. Basic Clin Pharmacol Toxicol. 2005;96(6):399–409.
33. Bonilla-Jaime H, Sánchez-Salcedo JA, Estevez-Cabrera MM, Molina-Jiménez T, Cortes-Altamirano JL, Alfaro-Rodríguez A. Depression and pain: use of antidepressants. Curr Neuropharmacol. 2022;20(2):384–402.
34. Moore RA, Derry S, Aldington D, Cole P, Wiffen PJ. Amitriptyline for neuropathic pain in adults. Cochrane Database Syst Rev. 2015;2015:7.
35. Seetharaman J, Poddar U, Yachha SK, Srivastava A, Sen Sarma M. Efficacy of amitriptyline in pediatric functional abdominal pain disorders: a randomized placebo-controlled trial. J Gastroenterol Hepatol. 2022;37(4):685–91.
36. Derry S, Wiffen PJ, Aldington D, Moore RA. Nortriptyline for neuropathic pain in adults. Cochrane Database Syst Rev. 2015;1(1):CD011209.
37. Kremer M, Salvat E, Muller A, Yalcin I, Barrot M. Antidepressants and gabapentinoids in neuropathic pain: mechanistic insights. Neuroscience. 2016;338:183–206.
38. Chen J, Li L, Shao-Rui C, Chen H, Jing-Dun X, Sirrieh RE, MacLean DM, Zhang Y, Meng-Hua Z, Jayaraman V, Pan HL. The a2d-1-NMDA receptor complex is critically involved in neuropathic pain development and gabapentin therapeutic actions. Cell Rep. 2018;22:2307–21.
39. Chincholkar M. Analgesic mechanisms of gabapentinoids and effects in experimental pain models: a narrative review. Br J Anaesth. 2018;120(6):1315–34.
40. Wiffen PJ, Derry S, Bell RF, et al. Gabapentin for chronic neuropathic pain in adults. Cochrane Database Syst Rev. 2017;6(6):CD007938.
41. Giménez-Campos MS, Pimenta-Fermisson-Ramos P, Díaz-Cambronero JI, Carbonell-Sanchís R, López-Briz E, Ruíz-García V. A systematic review and meta-analysis of the effectiveness and adverse events of gabapentin and pregabalin for sciatica pain. Aten Primaria. 2022;54(1):102144.
42. Lambru G, Zakrzewska J, Matharu M. Trigeminal neuralgia: a practical guide. Pract Neurol. 2021;21(5):392–402.
43. Wiffen PJ, Derry S, Lunn MPT, Moore RA. Topiramate for neuropathic pain and fibromyalgia in adults. Cochrane Database Syst Rev. 2013;2013(8):CD008314.
44. Zar-Kessler CAM, Belkind-Gerson J, Bender S, Kuo BM. Treatment of functional abdominal pain with antidepressants: benefits, adverse effects, and the gastroenterologist's role. J Pediatr Gastroenterol Nutr. 2017;65(1):16–21.
45. Bonilla S, Nurko S. Focus on the use of antidepressants to treat pediatric functional abdominal pain: current perspectives. Clin Exp Gastroenterol. 2018;11:365–72.
46. Siracusa R, Paola RD, Cuzzocrea S, Impellizzeri D. Fibromyalgia: pathogenesis, mechanisms, diagnosis and treatment options update. Int J Mol Sci. 2021;22(8):3891.
47. Patetsos E, Horjales-Araujo E. Treating chronic pain with SSRIs: what do we know? Pain Res Manag. 2016;2016:2020915.
48. Cohen SP, Mao J. Neuropathic pain: mechanisms and their clinical implications. BMJ. 2014;348:f7656.
49. Gül ŞK, Tepetam H, Gül HL. Duloxetine and pregabalin in neuropathic pain of lung cancer patients. Brain Behav. 2020;10(3):e01527.

50. Tanenberg RJ, Irving GA, Risser RC, et al. Duloxetine, pregabalin, and duloxetine plus gabapentin for diabetic peripheral neuropathic pain management in patients with inadequate pain response to gabapentin: an open-label, randomized, noninferiority comparison. Mayo Clin Proc. 2011;86(7):615–26.
51. Kamata M, Naito S, Higuchi H, Suzuki A, Otani K. Efficacy of milnacipran in the treatment of chronic pain syndromes. Int J Psychiatry Clin Pract. 2010;14(1):68–71.
52. Soleimanpour H, Imani F, Dolati S, Soleimanpour M, Shahsavarinia K. Management of pain using magnesium sulphate: a narrative review. Postgrad Med. 2022;134(3):260–6.
53. Urits I, Jung JW, Amgalan A, et al. Utilization of magnesium for the treatment of chronic pain. Anesth Pain Med. 2021;11(1):e112348.
54. Morel V, Pickering ME, Goubayon J, Djobo M, Macian N, Pickering G. Magnesium for pain treatment in 2021? State of the art. Nutrients. 2021;13(5):1397.
55. Borgeat A, Wilder-Smith OH, Saiah M, Rifat K. Subhypnotic doses of propofol possess direct antiemetic properties. Anesth Analg. 1992;74(4):539–41.
56. Celik M, Dostbil A, Aksoy M, Ince I, Ahiskalioglu A, Comez M, Erdem AF. Is infusion of subhypnotic propofol as effective as dexamethasone in prevention of postoperative nausea and vomiting related to laparoscopic cholecystectomy? A randomized controlled trial. Biomed Res Int. 2015;2015:349806.
57. Yalcin EK, Kim D, Mao G, Rivas E, Markwei M, Chahar P, Keebler A, Cywinski JB, Kurz A, Turan A. Effect of intraoperative subhypnotic infusion of propofol on postoperative nausea and vomiting: a retrospective analysis. J Clin Anesth. 2022;78:110672.
58. Grant MC, Kim J, Page AJ, Hobson D, Wick E, Wu CL. The effect of intravenous midazolam on postoperative nausea and vomiting: a meta-analysis. Anesth Analg. 2016;122(3):656–63.
59. Rizk MK, Tolba R, Kapural L, Mitchell J, Lopez R, Mahboobi R, Vrooman B, Mekhail N. Differential epidural block predicts the success of visceral block in patients with chronic visceral abdominal pain. Pain Pract. 2012;12(8):595–601.
60. Karolina Budych K, Helms T, Schultz C. How do patients with rare diseases experience the medical encounter? Exploring role behavior and its impact on patient-physician interaction. Health Policy. 2012;105(2-3):154–64.

Chapter 10
Open Surgical Approach for Median Arcuate Ligament Syndrome: Technical Considerations

Melinda S. Schaller and Manju Kalra

History of the Open Surgical Approach

In most individuals, the diaphragmatic crura form a fibrous arch, which passes superior to the celiac trunk as they decussate to form the ventral border of the aortic hiatus. This structure is known as the median arcuate ligament (MAL). However, in 3–24% of people, the MAL is located anterior to the celiac trunk, causing compression [1–4]. In a fraction of these individuals, this compression becomes symptomatic. The first published case of open surgical treatment of symptomatic compression of the celiac axis was from Harjola in 1963 [5]. Over the next decade, several small series and case reports were published by his group and others [6–8]. In 1985, Reilly reported the largest open operative series to date and described preoperative characteristics which were most predictive of postoperative symptomatic improvement, and those included postprandial pain, age between 40 and 60 years, and weight loss of 20 or more pounds [9]. Interestingly, Reilly found that the greatest symptomatic improvement occurred in those individuals who had both celiac axis decompression and an operative technique that ensured celiac patency, such as dilation or reconstruction [9]. In the nearly 40 years since, operative strategies have evolved to include open decompression with ganglionectomy, often without arterial reconstruction, as well as laparoscopic and robotic decompression [10, 11].

M. S. Schaller (✉) · M. Kalra
Division of Vascular and Endovascular Surgery, Mayo Clinic, Rochester, MN, USA
e-mail: schaller.melinda@mayo.edu; kalra.manju@mayo.edu

D. Shouhed et al. (eds.), *Median Arcuate Ligament Syndrome*,
https://doi.org/10.1007/978-3-031-80740-4_10

Preoperative and Anesthesia Considerations

Once the decision has been made to proceed with an open release of the MAL, the patient should be evaluated for surgical fitness. As many of these patients are young and otherwise healthy, an extensive preoperative evaluation is typically unnecessary. One should consider obtaining preoperative blood work, including markers of nutritional status, depending on how limited oral intake has been. Prior to commencing the operation, the preoperative cross-sectional imaging should be reviewed to confirm any aberrant arterial anatomy, such as a replaced/accessory left hepatic artery.

The procedure is performed under general anesthesia. An epidural catheter can be a useful adjunct in patients who have required multimodal pain regimens preoperatively. An orogastric tube should be placed to assist with identifying the esophagus during exposure to the supraceliac aorta.

Operative Technique

The procedure is performed via an upper midline incision from the xiphoid to approximately 2 cm cephalad to the umbilicus. The intraperitoneal space should be evaluated for any unexpected findings. The surgeon should then confirm the appropriate placement of the orogastric tube via palpation. The left lobe of the liver is mobilized by division of the left triangular ligament. Next, the gastrohepatic ligament is palpated to evaluate for a pulse to indicate an aberrant left hepatic artery. If an accessory left hepatic artery is present, determined from preoperative imaging, this can be ligated without concern. Should a replaced left hepatic artery be present, all attempts should be made to preserve the artery, such as dissecting along its length to allow for increased mobility. While most retrospective reviews regarding replaced left hepatic artery ligation have demonstrated no significant negative postoperative outcomes, there have been isolated reports of hepatic necrosis following ligation [12–14]. The gastrohepatic ligament is then divided. A fixed retractor, such as the Omni, is placed to retract the liver to the right, the stomach to the left, and the colon caudally. The supraceliac aorta is then palpated. The crura overlying the aorta are divided with electrocautery. This is the "endpoint" for division of the MAL (Fig. 10.1).

The hepatic artery is next identified via palpation and is circumferentially dissected. The hepatic artery is cleared of surrounding neuronal tissue as the artery is dissected in a distal to proximal orientation. This allows a safe approach to the celiac trunk and its branches. Once the celiac truck is identified, the splenic and left gastric arteries are similarly dissected free from enveloping neuronal tissue (Fig. 10.2). The left gastric artery can be ligated without clinical consequence if the surgeon believes it will allow for better exposure, although we have not found this to be necessary in our practice. The dense MAL is then divided proceeding from the

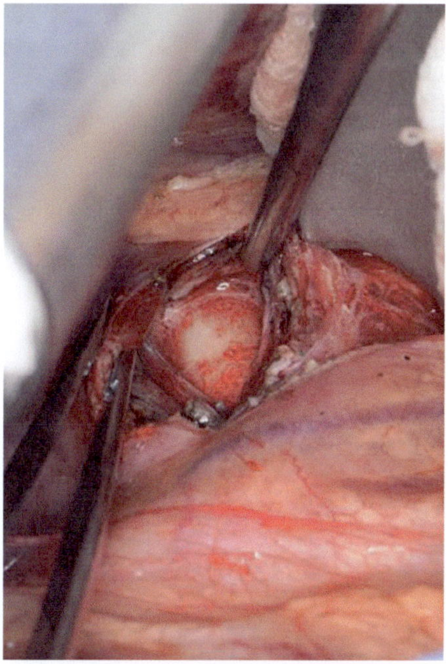

Fig. 10.1 Supraceliac aortic exposure

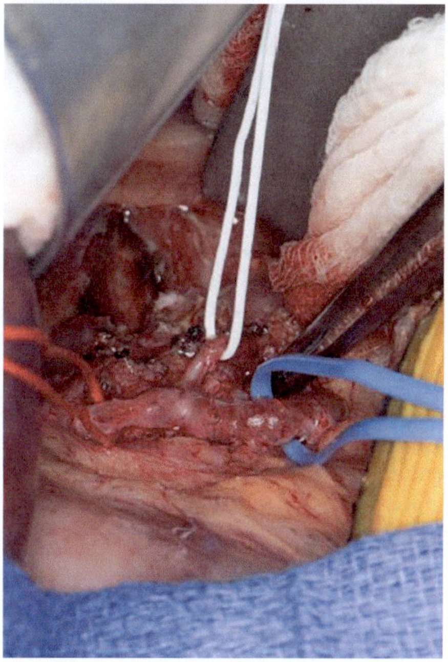

Fig. 10.2 Celiac trunk and branches. The red loop is around the common hepatic artery, the blue loop is around the splenic artery, and the white loop is around the left gastric artery

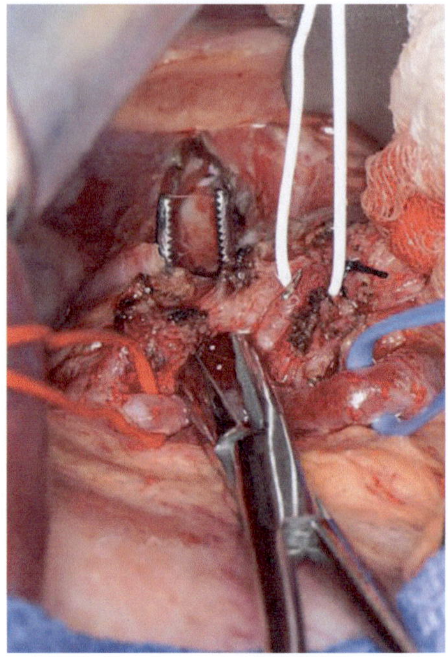

Fig. 10.3 Division of the median arcuate ligament proceeding from the celiac trunk exposure to the supraceliac aortic exposure

celiac truck exposure to the prior supraceliac aortic exposure (Fig. 10.3). The surgeon must be sure to skeletonize the celiac trunk, performing a thorough neurolysis. The celiac ganglion on either side of the celiac truck are then resected, including surrounding crural muscle fibers. The ganglia appear as irregular masses in the retroperitoneum, with the left often being larger and more well-defined than the right [1]. We believe that MALS represents a primary neurogenic pain disorder from compression of the splanchnic nerve plexus, so resection of nerve fibers and the ganglion is crucial [15, 16].

The surgeon must then determine if vascular reconstruction is necessary. The celiac artery is inspected, and patency is assessed via palpation. A sterile Doppler or an intraoperative ultrasound can be used to assist with decision-making. With the encouraging outcomes associated with laparoscopic and robotic MAL release, we have shifted our practice away from vascular reconstruction. In our practice, vascular reconstruction is typically reserved for those individuals with proven celiac trunk occlusion after MAL release. Should a vascular reconstruction be considered, options include a patch angioplasty of the celiac trunk, an aorto-celiac bypass, or arterial resection and primary end-to-end anastomosis in cases of celiac artery elongation. The short-term outcomes, as well as the long-term freedom from treatment failure, between open and laparoscopic approaches to MAL decompression and ganglionectomy have been reported to be very similar in multiple series [10, 11, 17].

Postoperative Care

The orogastric tube is removed at the conclusion of the operation. Patients are admitted to the hospital post-operatively on a general surgical floor. Should the patient not experience postoperative nausea, sips of liquids can be started on the evening of surgery and the diet can advance as tolerated. Patients can be dismissed from the hospital once they are tolerating a regular diet and postoperative pain is controlled on an oral regimen. If a vascular reconstruction was not performed, no additional imaging is needed at follow-up. We do not routinely order postoperative imaging as we believe MALS represents a primary neurogenic pain disorder. Typically, patients are seen back for a postoperative visit 4–6 weeks following the operation. Any additional follow-up can be scheduled on a case-by-case basis. We tend to counsel patients regarding the relative high rates of symptom recurrence and recommend that they contact our office should their symptoms reoccur.

References

1. Lindner HH, Kemprud E. A clinicoanatomical study of the arcuate ligament of the diaphragm. Arch Surg. 1971;103(5):600–5. https://doi.org/10.1001/archsurg.1971.01350110102016.
2. Petnys A, Puech-Leão P, Zerati AE, et al. Prevalence of signs of celiac axis compression by the median arcuate ligament on computed tomography angiography in asymptomatic patients. J Vasc Surg. 2018;68(6):1782–7. https://doi.org/10.1016/j.jvs.2018.04.044.
3. Derrick JR, Pollard HS, Moore RM. The pattern of arteriosclerotic narrowing of the celiac and superior mesenteric arteries. Ann Surg. 1959;149(5):684–9. https://doi.org/10.1097/00000658-195905000-00009.
4. Park CM, Chung JW, Kim HB, Shin SJ, Park JH. Celiac axis stenosis: incidence and etiologies in asymptomatic individuals. Korean J Radiol. 2001;2(1):8–13. https://doi.org/10.3348/kjr.2001.2.1.8.
5. Harjola PT. A rare obstruction of the coeliac artery. Report of a case. Ann Chir Gynaecol Fenn. 1963;52:547–50.
6. Harjola PT, Lahtiharju A. Celiac axis syndrome. Abdominal angina caused by external compression of the celiac artery. Am J Surg. 1968;115(6):864–9. https://doi.org/10.1016/0002-9610(68)90537-0.
7. Snyder MA, Mahoney EB, Rob CG. Symptomatic celiac artery stenosis due to constriction by the neurofibrous tissue of the celiac ganglion. Surgery. 1967;61(3):372–6.
8. Dunbar JD, Molnar W, Beman FF, Marable SA. Compression of the celiac trunk and abdominal angina. Am J Roentgenol Radium Therapy, Nucl Med. 1965;95(3):731–44. https://doi.org/10.2214/ajr.95.3.731.
9. Reilly LM, Ammar AD, Stoney RJ, Ehrenfeld WK. Late results following operative repair for celiac artery compression syndrome. J Vasc Surg. 1985;2(1):79–91.
10. Jimenez JC, Harlander-Locke M, Dutson EP. Open and laparoscopic treatment of median arcuate ligament syndrome. J Vasc Surg. 2012;56(3):869–73. https://doi.org/10.1016/j.jvs.2012.04.057.
11. DeCarlo C, Woo K, van Petersen AS, et al. Factors associated with successful median arcuate ligament release in an international, multi-institutional cohort. J Vasc Surg. 2023;77(2):567–577.e2. https://doi.org/10.1016/j.jvs.2022.10.022.

12. Ang RRG, Lee HJ, Bae JS, et al. Safety of ligation of aberrant left hepatic artery originating from left gastric artery in laparoscopic gastrectomy for gastric cancer. Sci Rep. 2020;10(1):5856. https://doi.org/10.1038/s41598-020-62587-7.
13. Tao W, Peng D, Cheng YX, Zhang W. Clinical significance of aberrant left hepatic artery during gastrectomy: a systematic review. World J Clin Cases. 2022;10(10):3121–30. https://doi.org/10.12998/wjcc.v10.i10.3121.
14. Yamamoto M, Zaima M, Yamamoto H, et al. Liver necrosis shortly after pancreaticoduodenectomy with resection of the replaced left hepatic artery. World J Surg Oncol. 2017;15(1):77. https://doi.org/10.1186/s12957-017-1151-2.
15. Skeik N, Cooper LT, Duncan AA, Jabr FI. Median arcuate ligament syndrome: a nonvascular, vascular diagnosis. Vasc Endovasc Surg. 2011;45(5):433–7. https://doi.org/10.1177/1538574411406453.
16. Chaum M, Shouhed D, Kim S, Walts AE, Marchevsky AM. Clinico-pathologic findings in patients with median arcuate ligament syndrome (celiac artery compression syndrome). Ann Diagn Pathol. 2021;52:151732. https://doi.org/10.1016/j.anndiagpath.2021.151732.
17. Chen AJ, Yeh S, Dhindsa Y, Lawrence PF, Woo K. Outcomes of median arcuate ligament release: a single institution retrospective review. Ann Vasc Surg. 2023;94:296–300. https://doi.org/10.1016/j.avsg.2023.02.030.

Chapter 11
Laparoscopic Median Arcuate Ligament Release: Technical Aspects for a Safe and Effective Procedure

Amanda Belluzzi, Kamal Abi Mosleh, and Omar M. Ghanem

Introduction

The surgical management of median arcuate ligament syndrome (MALS) targets both the vascular and neurogenic elements of the condition. The goals of this procedure are to alleviate the physical compression on the celiac trunk and to conduct a neurolysis and/or neurectomy of the celiac ganglion fibers. The laparoscopic surgical approach for MAL release was initially described by Roayaie et al. in 2000 [1], and its utilization has steadily increased over the past two decades. According to a nationwide analysis by Kroh et al., the adoption of the laparoscopic approach increased from 2010 to 2020, with 22% of all MAL release procedures employing this method by the end of the study period [2]. This surge can be attributed in part to the growing evidence published during this period, supporting laparoscopic MAL release as a safe and effective procedure with excellent, cost-effective postoperative symptomatic resolution [3].

While earlier studies showed no disparities in postoperative outcomes between the open and laparoscopic techniques [4], current research has consistently demonstrated the superior benefits of the laparoscopic approach. These include reduced intraoperative and postoperative complications, faster recovery times, lower hospital costs, decreased readmission rates, and improved immediate and long-term symptom relief [5–13]. The open technique reported a higher rate of major complications (4.0% vs. 0.5%) and a longer hospital stay than the laparoscopic approach

A. Belluzzi · K. A. Mosleh
Department of Metabolic and Abdominal Wall Reconstructive Surgery, Mayo Clinic, Rochester, MN, USA
e-mail: abimosleh.kamal@mayo.edu

O. M. Ghanem (✉)
Department of Surgery, Mayo Clinic, Rochester, MN, USA
e-mail: ghanem.omar@mayo.edu

D. Shouhed et al. (eds.), *Median Arcuate Ligament Syndrome*,
https://doi.org/10.1007/978-3-031-80740-4_11

[2]. It is essential, however, to acknowledge potential limitations with the laparoscopic method, such as challenges in controlling bleeding sources, the risk of incomplete compression release, and a higher likelihood of injury to major vascular landmarks during blunt laparoscopic dissection. Additionally, cases of persistent celiac trunk compression may necessitate revisional operations like endovascular angioplasty, stenting, or even conversion to open surgery with vascular reconstruction [14].

When examining the merits and limitations of the laparoscopic and robotic approaches, limited data come from a single institutional series and the superiority of one over the other cannot be established [2]. Some studies suggest that both laparoscopic and robotic-assisted techniques are relatively comparable, with the only limitation in the laparoscopic approach being the requirement for more skilled assistant proficiency [3]. On the other hand, concerns regarding the robotic-assisted technique include the absence of haptic feedback compared to straight-stick laparoscopy with finer instrument tips, along with a prolonged time to hemorrhage control in case of vascular injury when compared to the already disadvantaged laparoscopic technique [15].

Surgical Technique

The procedure begins with the patient in the supine position, and their lower extremities adducted. The optimal technique for achieving pneumoperitoneum and accessing the peritoneal cavity is still a subject of debate. This can be achieved in a variety of ways, either directly under vision using an optical 5-mm trocar, by introducing a Veress needle 2 cm below the left costal margin in the midclavicular line, or even using an open technique in some cases [1, 5, 8, 16–21]. The surgical table is then inclined in a 30° reverse Trendelenburg position.

In the majority of instances, the laparoscopic MAL release procedure utilizes a total of four trocars [1, 5, 8, 9, 13, 18, 22, 23]. Once the abdomen is insufflated with carbon dioxide to a pressure of 12–15 mmHg, the remaining four ports are placed under direct visualization. These ports include (Fig. 11.1):

(a) A 5-mm working port.
(b) A 10-mm 45° camera port, approximately 8 cm from the xyphoid for optimal visualization.
(c) A 10-mm left midclavicular line working port in the upper quadrant for dissection.
(d) A 5- or 10-mm left anterior axillary line port under the left costal arch for the assistant [1, 18, 24].

The majority of inserted ports are situated relatively high up in the abdomen, with the lowest being the camera port positioned about 8 cm inferior to the xyphoid. This placement is intentional, aiming to get the best view of the celiac ganglion

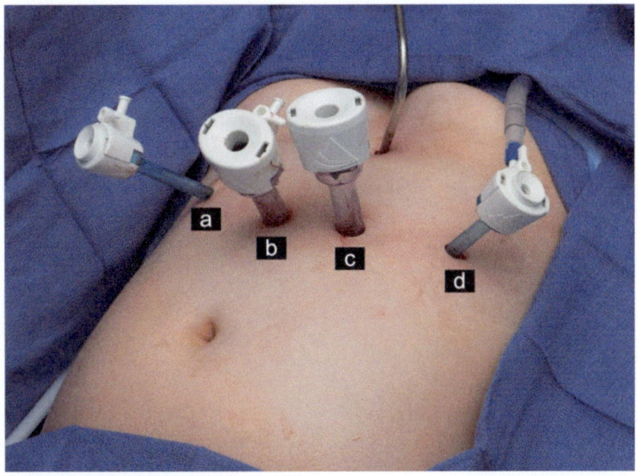

Fig. 11.1 Trocar placement sites

during dissection. The 12-mm port is typically positioned on the right-hand side to facilitate prompt suturing with a polypropylene thread in the event of bleeding.

At the beginning of every case, two 5–0 polypropylene threads, cut to approximately 17 cm in length, must be readily available in anticipation of potential bleeding, given the limited time for intervention. Following a thorough inspection of the peritoneal cavity to ensure the absence of injury or bleeding, the pars flaccida of the hepatogastric ligament is accessed to identify the origin of the common hepatic artery (CHA) from the celiac trunk. If the CHA lymph nodes are sizable, they are typically dissected to obtain proper access to the nerve bundles above the artery. Special attention is required for the lymphatic ductules between the common hepatic and celiac arteries, as chyle leakage can be effectively managed with superficial polypropylene sutures. It is important to note that injuries to the esophagus and celiac trunk have been documented, along with cases of postoperative superinfection of chylous cysts following celiac trunk exposure [25]. In cases with extensive adhesions from previous surgeries, meticulous adhesiolysis may be necessary to optimize exposure during the dissection. Subsequently, the surgeon can commence the dissection of nerve fibers down to the level of the adventitia, extending backward to the trifurcation of the celiac artery and the origin of the left gastric artery (Fig. 11.2). Then, exposure of the proximal segment of the splenic artery is performed to confirm the current location at the trifurcation. This step also facilitates navigating around the left gastric artery as closely to its base as possible (Fig. 11.3). Following this plane posteriorly toward the base of the right crus reveals the correct and ideal plane for the MAL release. At this point, the laparoscopic right angle is utilized to encircle the left gastric artery and facilitate the placement of a vessel loop.

Next, the attention turns to identifying the appropriate plane for the MAL release. This involves employing blunt dissection alternating the use of a laparoscopic suction cannula unit and ultrasonic dissector until reaching the base of the celiac trunk. Traction is then applied to the vessel loop in the direction of the patient's left leg (Figs. 11.4 and 11.5). With the left gastric artery retracted downward, the

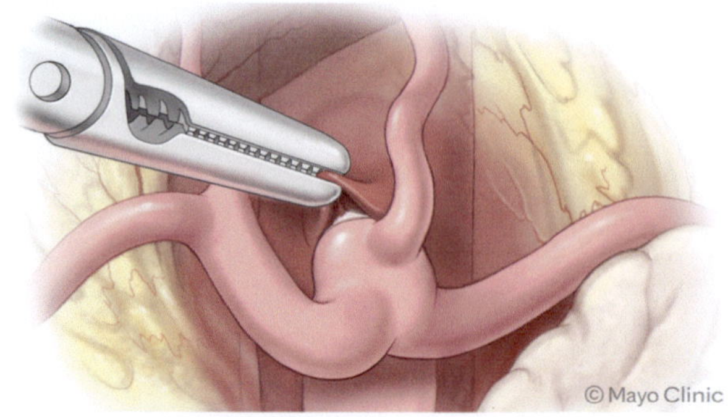

Fig. 11.2 Trifurcation of the celiac trunk with the left gastric artery, common hepatic artery, and splenic artery

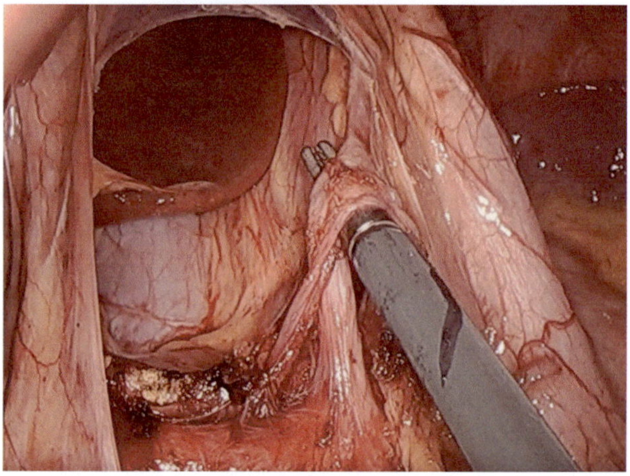

Fig. 11.3 Isolation of the left gastric artery

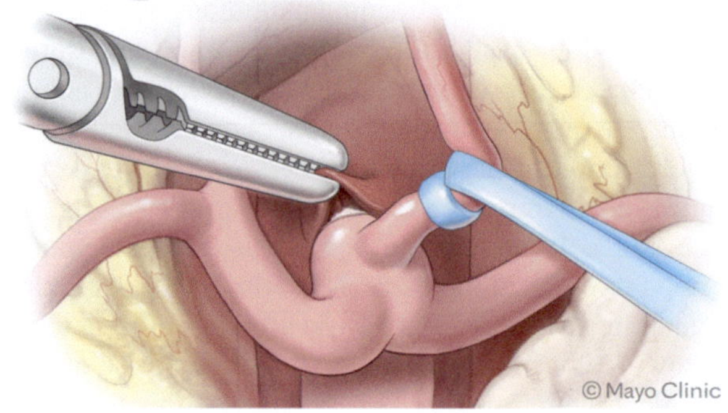

Fig. 11.4 Trifurcation with the left gastric artery (vessel loop) retracted downward

comprehensive dissection and exposure of the celiac trunk are accomplished using an L-hook cautery (Figs. 11.6 and 11.7).

The dissection of the MAL is then carried out by removing some fibers from the diaphragmatic crus where the aorta emerges and performing a lift test (Fig. 11.8). The dissection of MAL fibers is meticulously conducted in a layered fashion to

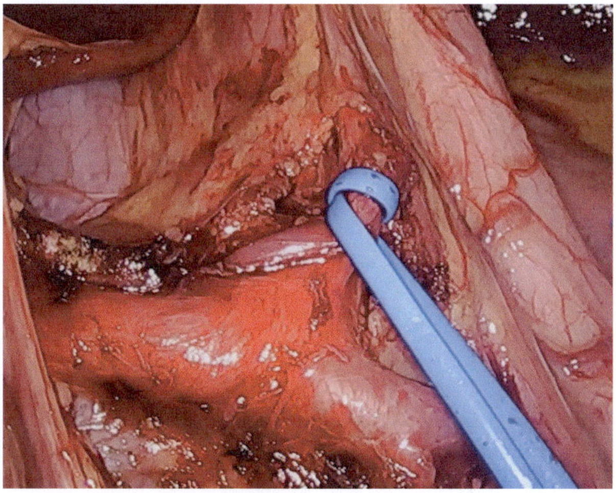

Fig. 11.5 Intraoperative image of vascular anatomy with a vessel loop seen retracting the left gastric in the direction of the left foot to increase exposure

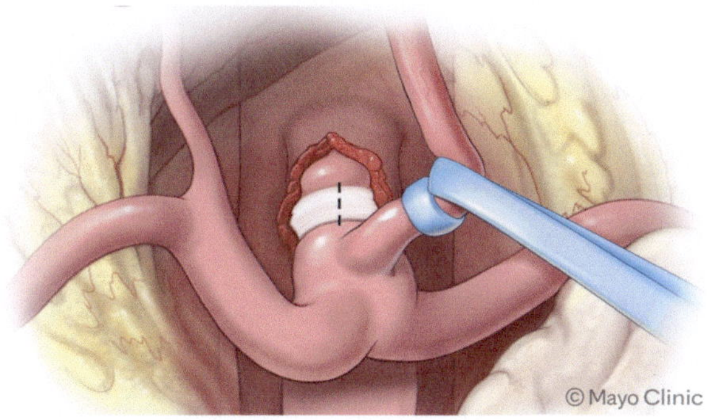

Fig. 11.6 Full exposure of the intact median arcuate ligament

prevent injury to the aorta. It is crucial at this juncture to be vigilant of branches of the phrenic artery that stem from the proximal celiac artery. Occasionally, bleeding can arise from an atypical position at 12 o'clock, rather than their usual lateral orientation, in a Y configuration within the MAL region. Such instances underscore the necessity of having a vascular surgeon readily available to swiftly manage any bleeding, potentially circumventing the need for transfusions. During the lift test, tension must consistently be directed away from the aorta to prevent potential damage from the heel of the hook cautery. Following this dissection, the suction cannula should be used to expose the aorta at least 3 cm cephalad to the origin of the celiac axis, ensuring the phrenic vessels and their branches remain undamaged (Figs. 11.9 and 11.10). While it is possible to sacrifice the phrenic artery on either side and securely clip both ends for optimal ligament exposure and dissection facilitation, it is generally not deemed necessary (Figs. 11.11 and 11.12). The final step of the procedure involves partially removing the celiac ganglion, typically not in its entirety to mitigate the risks of intraoperative lymphatic leaks associated with

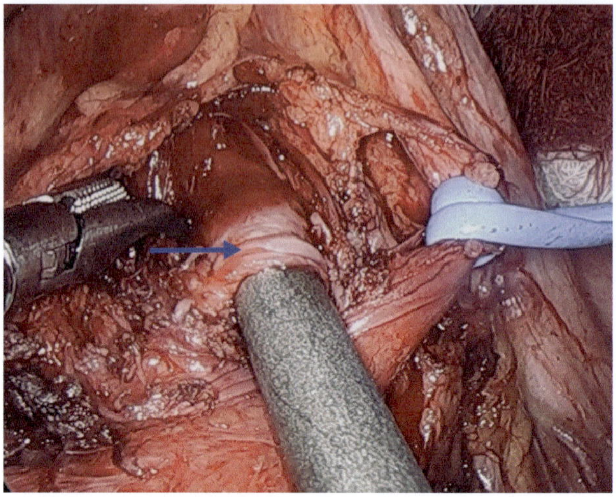

Fig. 11.7 Intraoperative image revealing the fully intact median arcuate ligament (arrow), with the suction device overlying the celiac trunk

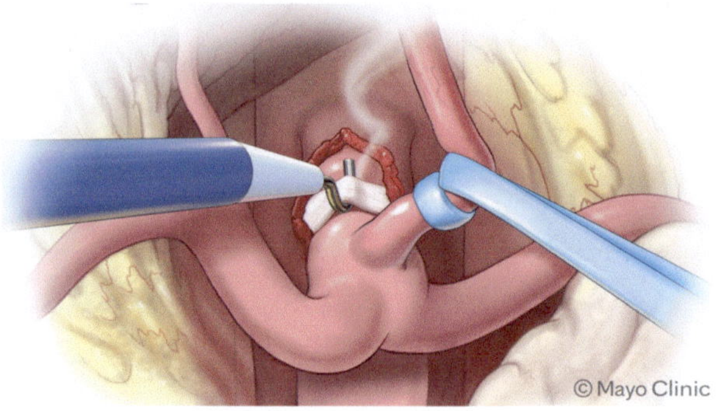

Fig. 11.8 Median arcuate ligament release, where fibers are divided by layers cutting through ligamentous, muscular, and neurovascular bundles

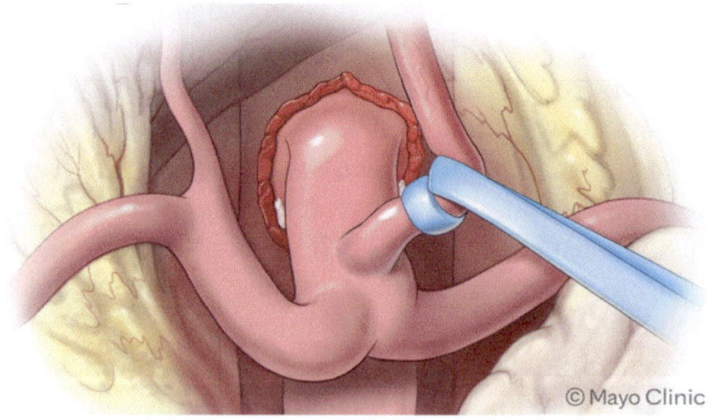

Fig. 11.9 Exposure of the aorta after median arcuate ligament release

aggressive dissection. The excised part of the celiac ganglion is sent for pathological examination.

Following the confirmation of hemostasis and a thorough examination of all vascular landmarks, the vessel loop encircling the left gastric artery is taken off, and a

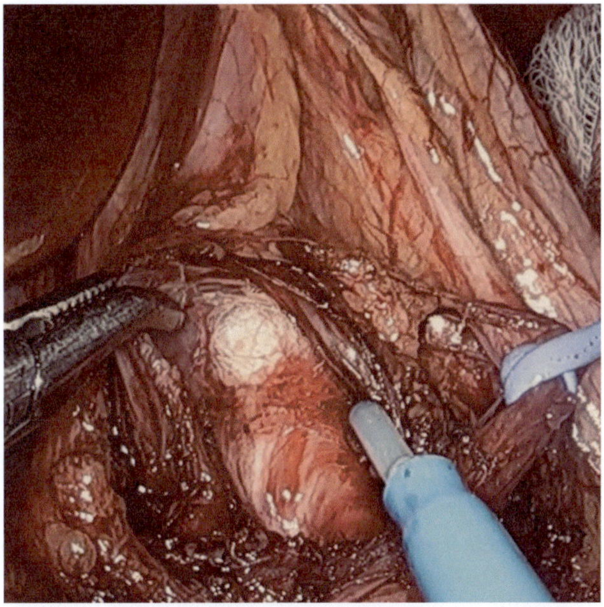

Fig. 11.10 Intraoperative image revealing the junction between the celiac trunk and the aorta, with the whitish appearance of the aorta apparent

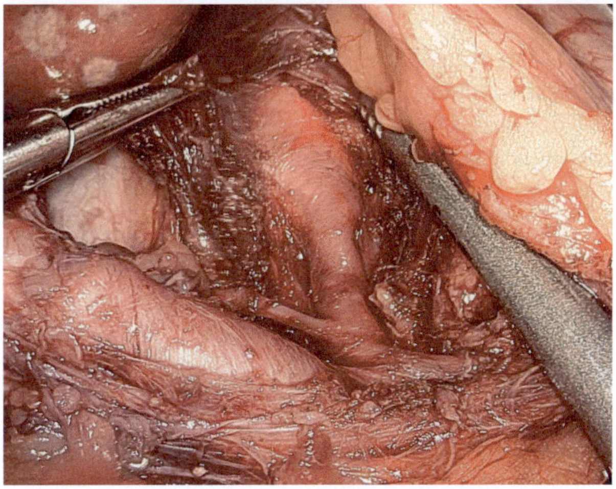

Fig. 11.11 Intraoperative image of fully exposed aorta and celiac trunk after median arcuate ligament release

gauze is positioned above the area. The abdomen is then deflated for approximately 10 min and then reinflated to confirm the absence of bleeding. Particular attention is directed toward securing control over any potential sources of bleeding, especially in the regions surrounding the dissected crural fibers. Any postoperative accumulation at the site requires vigilance, as it may lead to scarring and a recurrence of preoperative symptoms.

During the laparoscopic MAL release procedure, the use of intraoperative ultrasonography can be considered to evaluate the flow of the celiac artery after

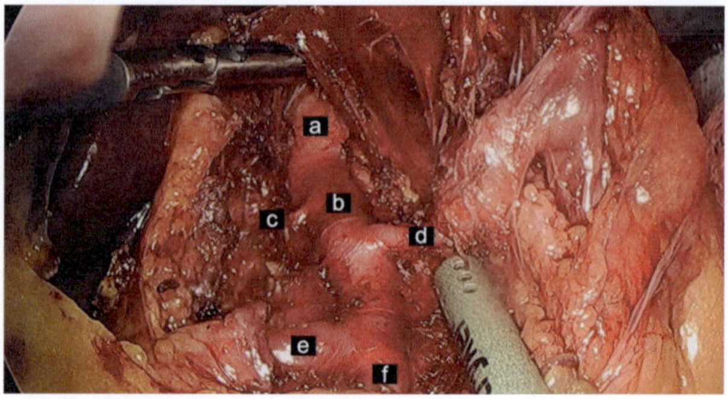

Fig. 11.12 Full exposure of vascular anatomy after median arcuate ligament release showing the a. abdominal aorta, b. celiac trunk, c. inferior phrenic artery, d. left gastric artery, e. common hepatic artery, and f. splenic artery

decompression. However, the decision to employ this technique is based on the surgeon's preference, as there is currently no consensus on its routine use. Some surgeons advocate for the evaluation of flow rate using intraoperative fluorescein angiography or ultrasonography, while others are in favor of simply visualizing adequate MAL release [1, 26–28]. In certain cases, intraoperative ultrasonography may not detect sufficient blood flow after the release, indicating a subset of patients that could potentially benefit from additional endovascular intervention [1].

Finally, all ports are removed under direct laparoscopic visualization, checking for any bleeding at the exit sites. The two 10-mm trocars are subsequently closed using absorbable synthetic braided sutures, along with the closure of all other incisions. The patient is extubated at the end of the procedure and discharged to the surgical ward. On the evening of the same day, the patient progresses to a clear liquid diet, with a further progression to solid food as tolerated. The following day, the patient is sent home with oral analgesics for pain relief, as needed, and can resume activities of daily living.

Conclusion

Laparoscopic MAL release is a safe and effective approach for the management of MALS in the hands of experienced surgeons. A thorough understanding of surgical anatomy and proper preoperative radiologic findings are paramount to mitigate complications and optimize clinical outcomes. The critical nature of the procedure necessitates that it be performed by surgeons who have received comprehensive training in minimally invasive techniques and in medical centers equipped with readily available multidisciplinary teams consisting of general, vascular, and pediatric surgeons, gastroenterologists, and radiologists.

References

1. Roayaie S, Jossart G, Gitlitz D, Lamparello P, Hollier L, Gagner M. Laparoscopic release of celiac artery compression syndrome facilitated by laparoscopic ultrasound scanning to confirm restoration of flow. J Vasc Surg. 2000;32(4):814–7.
2. Romero-Velez G, Barajas-Gamboa JS, Pantoja JP, et al. A nationwide analysis of median arcuate ligament release between 2010 and 2020: a NSQIP study. Surg Endosc. 2023;37(1):140–7.
3. Shin TH, Rosinski B, Strong A, Fayazzadeh H, Fathalizadeh A, Rodriguez J, El-Hayek K. Robotic versus laparoscopic median arcuate ligament (MAL) release: a retrospective comparative study. Surg Endosc. 2022;36(7):5416–23.
4. Jimenez JC, Harlander-Locke M, Dutson EP. Open and laparoscopic treatment of median arcuate ligament syndrome. J Vasc Surg. 2012;56(3):869–73.
5. San Norberto EM, Romero A, Fidalgo-Domingos LA, García-Saiz I, Taylor J, Vaquero C. Laparoscopic treatment of median arcuate ligament syndrome: a systematic review. Int Angiol. 2019;38(6):474–83.
6. DeCarlo C, Woo K, van Petersen AS, et al. Factors associated with successful median arcuate ligament release in an international, multi-institutional cohort. J Vasc Surg. 2023;77(2):567–77.e2
7. Metz FM, Blauw JTM, Brusse-Keizer M, Kolkman JJ, Bruno MJ, Geelkerken RH. Systematic review of the efficacy of treatment for median arcuate ligament syndrome. Eur J Vasc Endovasc Surg. 2022;64(6):720–32.
8. Cienfuegos JA, Estevez MG, Ruiz-Canela M, et al. Laparoscopic treatment of median arcuate ligament syndrome: analysis of long-term outcomes and predictive factors. J Gastrointest Surg. 2018;22(4):713–21.
9. Dowgiałło-Gornowicz N, Grochowska W, Lech P, Saluk S, Michalik M. Laparoscopic treatment of rare median arcuate ligament syndrome—medium-term follow-up. Pol Przegl Chir. 2021;93:25–9.
10. Kazmi SSH, Safi N, Berge ST, Kazmi M, Sundhagen JO, Hisdal J. Laparoscopic surgery for median arcuate ligament syndrome (MALS): a prospective cohort of 52 patients. Vasc Health Risk Manag. 2022;18:139–51.
11. Pather K, Kärkkäinen JM, Tenorio ER, et al. Long-term symptom improvement and health-related quality of life after operative management of median arcuate ligament syndrome. J Vasc Surg. 2021;73(6):2050–8.e4
12. Birkhold M, Khalifeh A, Nagarsheth K, Kavic SM. Median arcuate ligament syndrome is effectively relieved with minimally invasive surgery. JSLS. 2022;26:4.
13. Belluzzi A, Salame M, Abi Mosleh K, Rasmussen TE, Kendrick ML, Ghanem OM. Laparoscopic median arcuate ligament release: surgical technique and clinical outcomes. Surg Laparosc Endosc Percutan Tech. 2024;34(1):74–9. https://doi.org/10.1097/SLE.0000000000001257. PMID: 38190634.
14. Kim EN, Lamb K, Relles D, Moudgill N, DiMuzio PJ, Eisenberg JA. Median arcuate ligament syndrome-review of this rare disease. JAMA Surg. 2016;151(5):471–7.
15. Fernstrum C, Pryor M, Wright GP, Wolf AM. Robotic surgery for median arcuate ligament syndrome. JSLS. 2020;24:2.
16. Gülmez S, Aday U, Senger AS, Gündeş E. A new laparoscopic manoeuvre in median arcuate ligament syndrome. Balkan Med J. 2017;34(6):590–2.
17. De'Ath HD, Wong S, Szentpali K, Somers S, Peck T, Wakefield CH. The laparoscopic management of median arcuate ligament syndrome and its long-term outcomes. J Laparoendosc Adv Surg Tech A. 2018;28(11):1359–63.
18. Brody F, Richards NG. Median arcuate ligament release. J Am Coll Surg. 2014;219(4):e45–50.
19. El-Hayek KM, Titus J, Bui A, Mastracci T, Kroh M. Laparoscopic median arcuate ligament release: are we improving symptoms? J Am Coll Surg. 2013;216(2):272–9.
20. Wani S, Wakde V, Patel R, Patankar R, Mathur SK. Laparoscopic release of median arcuate ligament. J Minim Access Surg. 2012;8(1):16–8.

21. Nguyen T, Neale M, Lane R, Schiavone V, Samra JS, Hugh TJ. Laparoscopic management of the median arcuate ligament syndrome. ANZ J Surg. 2012;82(4):265–8.
22. Coelho JCU, Hosni AVE, Claus CM, Aguilera YSH, Abot GP, Freitas ATC, Costa M. Treatment of median arcuate ligament syndrome: outcome of laparoscopic approach. Arq Bras Cir Dig. 2020;33(1):e1495.
23. Baccari P, Civilini E, Dordoni L, Melissano G, Nicoletti R, Chiesa R. Celiac artery compression syndrome managed by laparoscopy. J Vasc Surg. 2009;50(1):134–9.
24. Do MV, Smith TA, Bazan HA, Sternbergh WC 3rd, Abbas AE, Richardson WS. Laparoscopic versus robot-assisted surgery for median arcuate ligament syndrome. Surg Endosc. 2013;27(11):4060–6.
25. Klimas A, Lemmer A, Bergert H, Brodhun M, Scholbach T, Großer K. Laparoscopic treatment of celiac artery compression syndrome in children and adolescents. Vasa. 2015;44(4):305–12.
26. Takach TJ, Livesay JJ, Reul GJ Jr, Cooley DA. Celiac compression syndrome: tailored therapy based on intraoperative findings. J Am Coll Surg. 1996;183(6):606–10.
27. Carbonell AM, Kercher KW, Heniford BT, Matthews BD. Multimedia article. Laparoscopic management of median arcuate ligament syndrome. Surg Endosc. 2005;19(5):729.
28. Vaziri K, Hungness ES, Pearson EG, Soper NJ. Laparoscopic treatment of celiac artery compression syndrome: case series and review of current treatment modalities. J Gastrointest Surg. 2009;13(2):293–8.

Chapter 12
Robotic Surgical Approach to Median Arcuate Ligament Syndrome: Technical Considerations Including Ganglion Resection

Jamie DeCicco, Peter Kanuika, Daniel Shouhed, and Kevin El-Hayek

Robotic Surgical Considerations

An early series of minimally invasive cases cautioned against the use of the robot due to the loss of haptic feedback in a case, which resulted in an aortic injury and conversion to open surgery [1], and others have shared this concern [2, 3]. Since this early experience with the robotic platform, multiple centers have demonstrated improved safety and efficacy with fewer to no conversions [4–7]. Table 12.1 provides a detailed list of the current published literature on robotic MALS including conversion rates and outcomes. With better knowledge of the anatomy and anatomical variants, improved technology, and more experience, conversions can be avoided almost completely. Additionally, with an increase in practice and comfort level, surgeons can adapt to the change in tactile feedback and appreciate improved visual

J. DeCicco (✉)
Cleveland Clinic Lerner College of Medicine of Case Western Reserve University, Cleveland, OH, USA

Division of General Surgery, Department of Surgery, The MetroHealth System, Cleveland, OH, USA

P. Kanuika
Department of Surgery, The MetroHealth System, Cleveland, OH, USA
e-mail: pkanuika@metrohealth.org

D. Shouhed
Robotic Surgical Institute of Southern California, Beverly Hills, CA, USA

K. El-Hayek
Department of Surgery, The MetroHealth System, Case Western Reserve University School of Medicine, Cleveland, OH, USA
e-mail: Kelhayek@metrohealth.org

D. Shouhed et al. (eds.), *Median Arcuate Ligament Syndrome*,
https://doi.org/10.1007/978-3-031-80740-4_12

Table 12.1 Review of the current robotic MALS literature

Author	Year	Study design	Patients	Mean follow-up (months)	Lost to follow-up	Ganglionectomy	Conversion rate	Complication rate	Symptom improvement
DeCicco [7]	2023	Retrospective cohort	36	9.3	1 (2.8%)	Yes	0%	3 (8.3%)	28 (77.8%)
Gerull [6]	2022	Retrospective cohort	74	12	12 (16.2%)	Nerve division	0%	3 (4.1%)	56 (75.6%)
Shin [8]	2022	Retrospective cohort	26	1.5	0	Nerve division	0%	0%	20 (76.9%)
Magnus [11]	2022	Retrospective cohort	9	22.7	0	No	0%	2 (22.2%)	8 (88.9%)
Fernstrum [4]	2020	Retrospective cohort	27	29.7	2 (7%)	Yes	2 (7%)	1 (4%)	18 (72%)
Khrucharoen [10]	2020	Retrospective cohort	18	15	0	Nerve division	1 (5.6%)	3 (16.7%)	14 (77.8%)
Bustos [14]	2020	Case report	1	5	0	Nerve division	0%	0%	1 (100%)
Thoolen [5]	2015	Retrospective cohort	9	5.8	0	Nerve division/ neurolysis	0%	0%	9 (100%)
Do [12]	2013	Retrospective cohort	4	20	0	Nerve division	0%	0%	2 (50%)
You [15]	2013	Case report	2	0.75	0	Yes	0%	0%	2 (100%)
Meyer [16]	2012	Case report	1	16	0	No	0%	0%	1 (100%)
Relles [17]	2012	Case series	3	11	0	Nerve division	0%	0%	2 (66.7%)
Jaik [18]	2007	Case report	1	1.3	0	No	0%	0%	1 (100%)

feedback having a stable camera with enhanced 3D vision and decreased tremor [7, 8].

The robot offers several technical advantages in this regard with a three-dimensional high-definition image, precise surgical movements around the aorta and celiac artery through enhanced articulation of instruments, and the addition of real-time augmented image guidance including ultrasound and indocyanine green (ICG) angiography. While the use of ultrasound and ICG angiography is available in all MIS, it is readily available and more easily integrated into the robotic platform without additional purchases, as is often the case for laparoscopic platforms. These benefits may allow for a more delicate and extensive dissection including celiac ganglionectomy and lymphadenectomy when compared to a completely laparoscopic approach [8]. There are also benefits to the patient using a minimally invasive approach (either laparoscopic or robotic), including decreased length of stay, decreased wound morbidity, decreased pain, faster recovery, and no compromise in patient outcomes [3, 7, 8].

Setup

To prepare for the operation, the patient is positioned appropriately in a supine position with a footboard, as steep reverse Trendelenburg is necessary for optimal access to the hiatus. A urinary catheter is optional, depending on the health status of the patient and the comfort level of the surgeon, as well as the team's proficiency. Additional anesthesia lines may be necessary depending on patient comorbidities and surgeon preference. Preoperative and anesthesia considerations are discussed in more detail in Chap. 13.

Entry to the peritoneal cavity for robotic MALS surgery can be achieved by any standard means; however, optimal entry at Palmer's point is favored by many minimally invasive surgeons. A total of four to five working trocars are ultimately placed across the abdomen—four 8-mm robotic ports and an optional 12-mm single bedside assistant port (Fig. 12.1). An open retractor with blades attached may be connected to the bed should conversion to an open procedure be required (Fig. 12.2a). A vascular tray and polypropylene sutures should be immediately available in case of bleeding and if rapid conversion is needed. A Kittner rolled gauze and/or Ray-tec sponge may be placed in the abdomen in case of bleeding and to maintain a bloodless field.

Patient positioning is critical for minimally invasive surgical techniques. A steep reverse-Trendelenburg position is necessary to maximize exposure of the foregut (Fig. 12.2a). This positioning is carried out prior to docking the DaVinci Robotic System (Intuitive, Sunnyvale, CA). A beside assistant can help guide robot docking (Fig. 12.2b). In arm 1 (left hand), a force or fenestrated bipolar forceps is often used, and a Maryland bipolar forceps can be exchanged for finer movements if needed. The camera is placed in arm 2. In arm 3, dissection is carried out with a monopolar permanent hook. Self-locking clips, scissors, and advanced energy devices can be

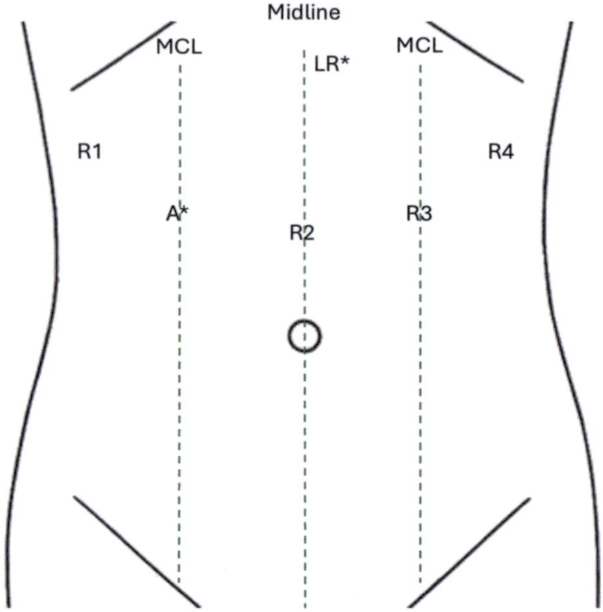

Fig. 12.1 Robotic arm positioning.
MCL = midclavicular line.
LR = liver retractor.
R1 = robotic arm 1.
A = assist port.
R2 = robotic arm 3.
R3 = robotic arm 3.
R4 = robotic arm 4.
*denotes optional site

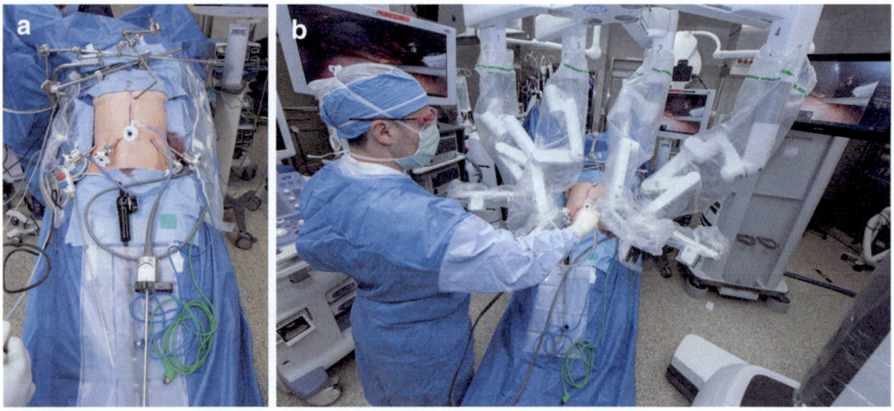

Fig. 12.2 (**a**) Patient in reverse Trendelenburg position with a setup including open retractor, liver retractor, assist port, and midline marking. (**b**) Beside assistant guiding robot docking

used in arm 3 if needed. In arm 4, a cadiere forceps or fenestrated prograsp is used for assistance. An assistant port is typically placed on the right side of the abdomen in the midclavicular line between arms 1 and 2 (Fig. 12.1). While optional, this port allows the bedside assistant to provide downward retraction, irrigation and suction, and passing of sutures and sponges throughout the case, as well as the ultrasound probe when utilizing intraoperative ultrasound (Fig. 12.2b). This site is also valuable for immediate bedside management of intraoperative bleeding such as pressure.

Surgical Technique

Once the robot is docked, the liver is retracted and gastrohepatic ligament exposed. Some surgeons prefer laparoscopic liver retractors (e.g., Nathanson retractor) placed under the left lateral hepatic lobe, while others achieve liver retraction from their bedside assistant. To eliminate the liver retractor incision, still others fashion a "hammock" with a Kittner rolled gauze and a self-locking suture, stitching the hammock to the anterior abdominal wall and retracting the left lateral hepatic lobe anteriorly to achieve exposure of the pars (Fig. 12.3). Next, the gastrohepatic ligament is divided to the level of the right diaphragmatic crus (Fig. 12.4). Prerelease ultrasound can be used to identify the median arcuate ligament and celiac artery takeoff under the right crus using the color/flow option (Fig. 12.5). The celiac takeoff diameter can be measured, demonstrating compression and limited blood flow through the artery.

Different approaches, including aortic, left gastric, or common hepatic artery approaches, can then be undertaken, depending on where the dissection begins. With an aortic approach, the right crus is dissected longitudinally from the base of the crus toward the anterior portion to expose the supraceliac aorta (Fig. 12.6). The crural incision is extended roughly 4–6 cm longitudinally. Retraction of the crus proceeds using traction and countertraction, with the bedside assistant providing caudal retraction of the celiac artery. Division of the right crus continues until the base of the celiac artery is reached (Fig. 12.7). Approaching the median arcuate ligament this way allows for the esophageal hiatus to remain intact and helps avoid injury to the underlying artery. After the division of the right crus, the fibrous bands of the median arcuate ligament are divided (Fig. 12.8). This area will eventually contain the celiac ganglion more distally along the celiac artery.

Care is taken to identify and dissect the common hepatic artery lymph node as part of the complete celiac lymphadenectomy. The inclusion of celiac

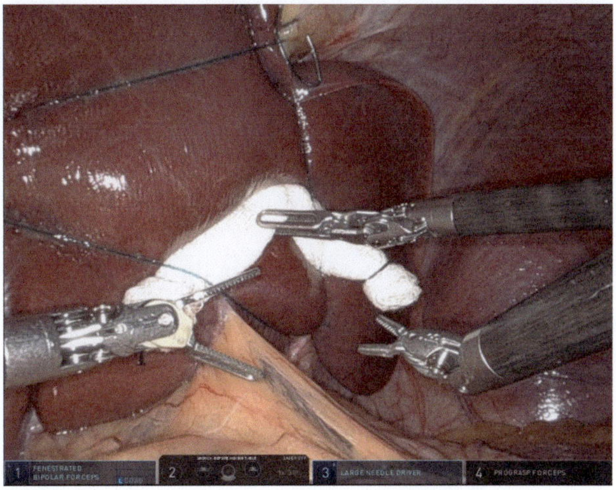

Fig. 12.3 Liver hammock with Kittner rolled gauze and self-locking suture to expose the pars flaccida of the gastrohepatic ligament and provide easier access to the right crus

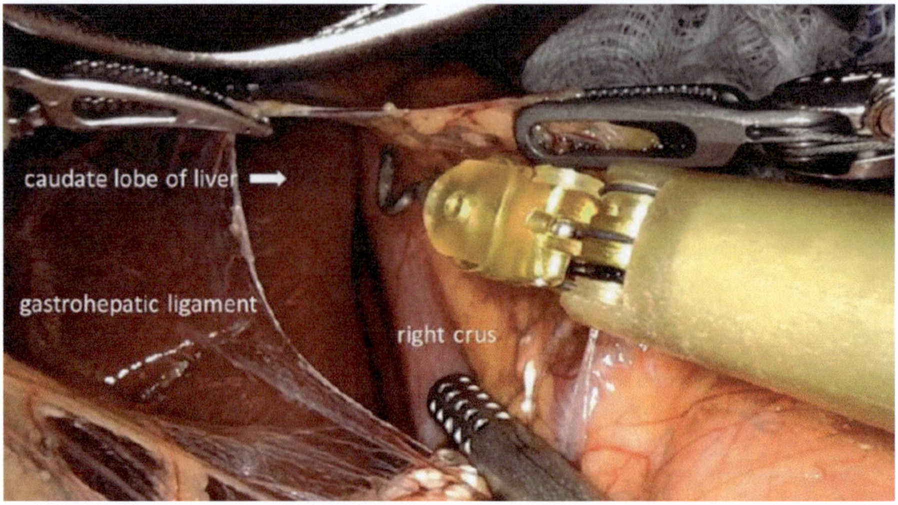

Fig. 12.4 Pars flaccida of the gastrohepatic ligament is divided to the level of the right diaphragmatic crus

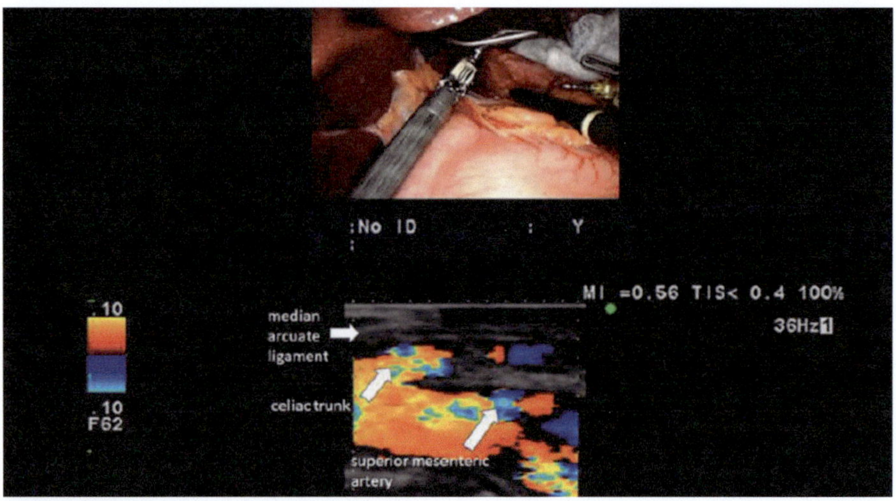

Fig. 12.5 Prerelease ultrasound identifies median arcuate ligament compression of the celiac artery

lymphadenectomy was described in the original operation during the open era [9]. Lymphadenectomy provides a greater guarantee of skeletonizing the vessels and, through analysis of these specimens, provides further insight into systemic pathology. As such, the authors recommend routine performance of lymphadenectomy, regardless of gross appearance, because non-grossly pathologic lymph nodes have been found to have pathologic findings upon specimen analysis [7]. The common hepatic artery is then traced to the takeoffs of the splenic and left gastric arteries,

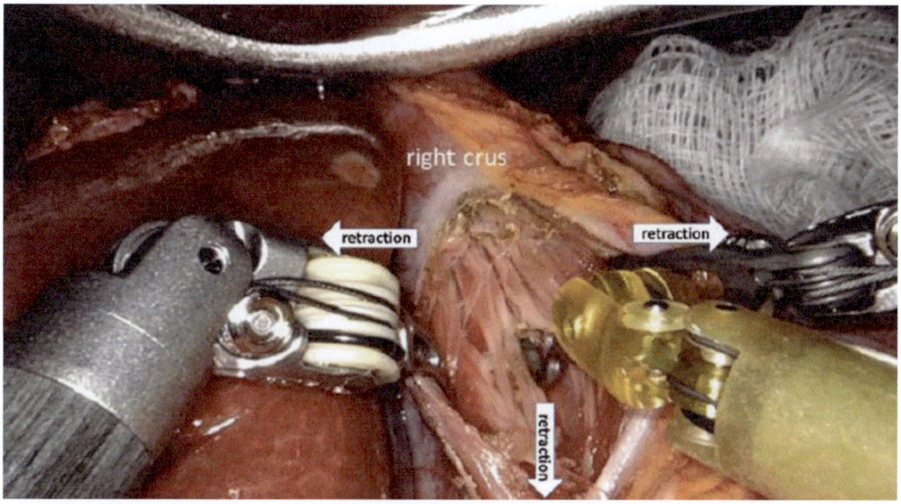

Fig. 12.6 Right crus longitudinal dissection starting at the base with retraction

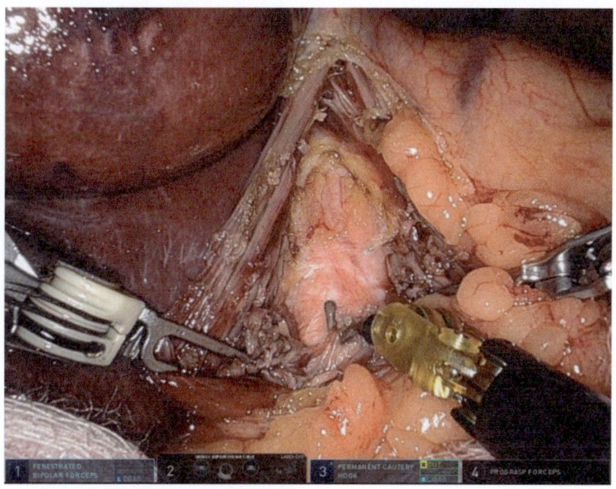

Fig. 12.7 Division of the right crus from its base up to the supraceliac aorta

identifying their common origins at the celiac artery. The lymphatic and nodal tissue dissection is carried through a place directly overlying the artery itself and is followed to the takeoff of the celiac artery, allowing complete division of the median arcuate ligament (Fig. 12.9). The celiac ganglion lies directly over the celiac artery, courses along the tributaries, and wraps 360 degrees around the abdominal aorta. To expose the celiac artery, the fibers of the celiac ganglion are completely divided and resected (Figs. 12.10 and 12.11). Using the electrocautery hook in an oblique fashion, each individual nerve fiber can be dissected free from the underlying artery and divided safely. This is done carefully to avoid arterial injury with the heel of the hook. The hook can be kept in view prior to applying energy with proper

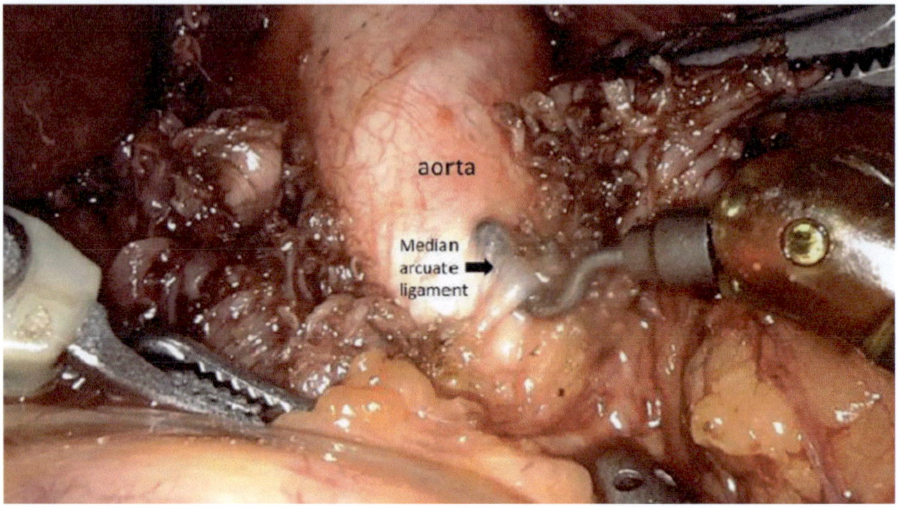

Fig. 12.8 Division of the median arcuate ligament

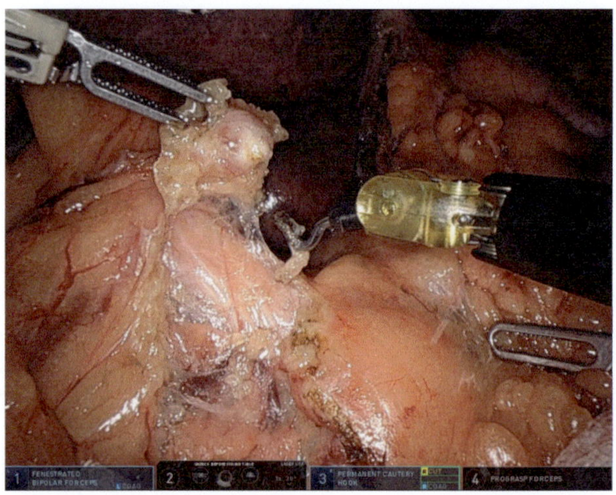

Fig. 12.9 Celiac lymphadenectomy of common hepatic artery lymph node

orientation. Skeletonization of common hepatic, left gastric, and splenic arteries for 180 degrees will help ensure complete release of vascular compression and complete anterior resection of the celiac ganglion (Fig. 12.12).

With the common hepatic artery or left gastric artery approach, dissection begins at the midpoint of the designated artery. Care should be taken not to travel too far distally on the left gastric artery as this can lead to inadvertent injury or division of the posterior vagus nerve. Care should also be taken not to dissect too far distally onto the common hepatic artery as this can lead to inadvertent injury to the cisterna chyli. Vessel loops around the left gastric artery and vein can be helpful in providing additional retraction and exposure. Following the course of the left gastric artery to

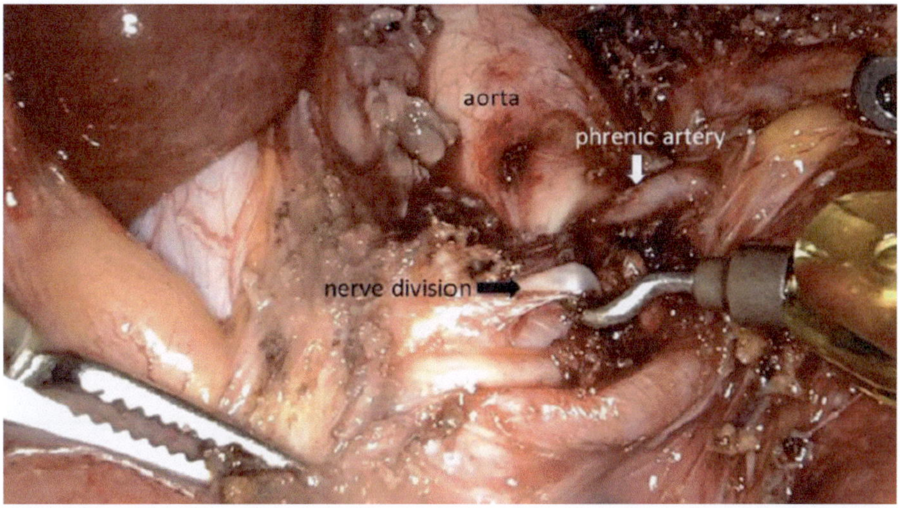

Fig. 12.10 Division of the celiac ganglia nerve fibers

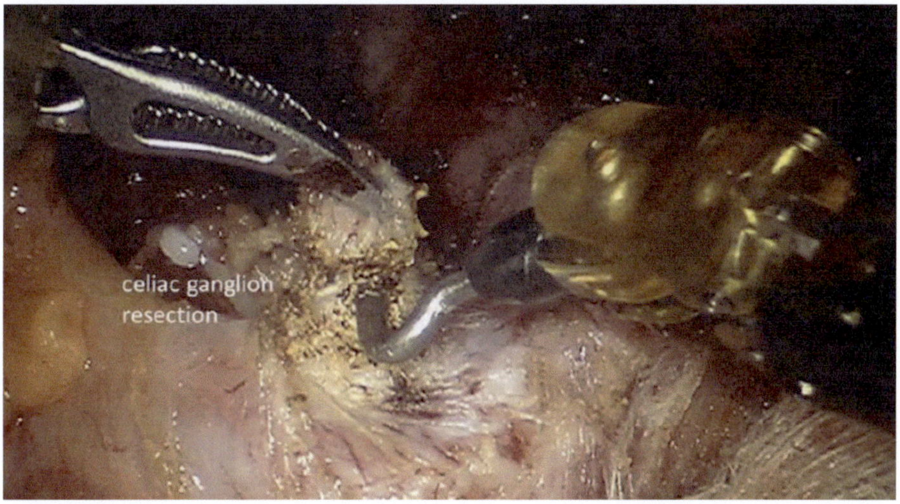

Fig. 12.11 Resection of the celiac ganglia

the common hepatic artery is a reliable method of finding the celiac artery. Once the celiac artery is identified, dissection can then be carried cephalad until the median arcuate ligament is found. Dissection then continues until the celiac artery is seen coming off the aorta. In difficult dissections, prior to dividing the median arcuate ligament, one can divert their attention to the base of the right crus and divide those muscle fibers to expose the aorta. Once the aorta and the distal aspect of the celiac artery are identified, joining those two areas will lead to proper release and

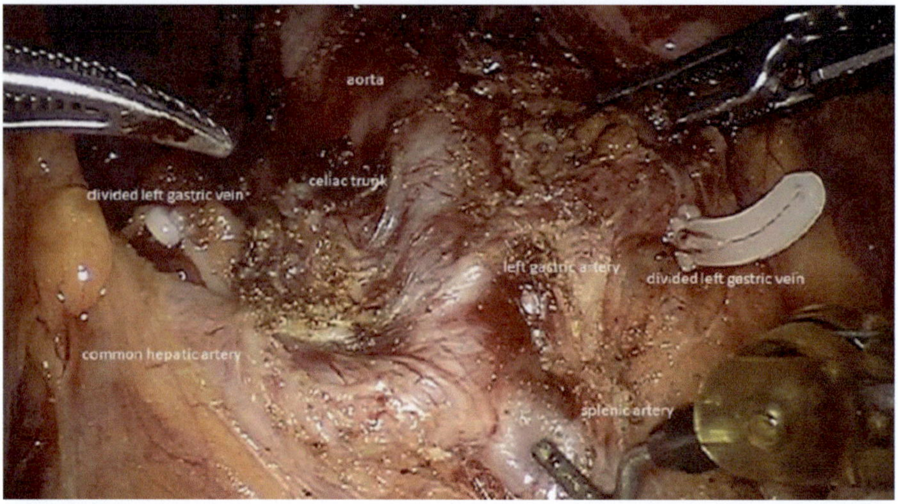

Fig. 12.12 Skeletonization of the celiac trunk and its tributaries for complete release and anterior resection

identification of the median arcuate ligament. The aortic approach more closely follows the principles of vascular surgery (i.e., "proximal control"), while advantages to the left gastric or common hepatic artery approach include additional preservation of the crural fibers.

To confirm adequate release, celiac patency can be assessed with intraoperative imaging. Post-release ultrasound can be employed to confirm no additional median arcuate ligament tissue above the celiac artery and quantify the anatomic resolution of the compression by noting an increase in the diameter of the celiac ostia as well as visualizing flow with color doppler (Fig. 12.13). Indocyanine green can also be administered intravenously with the performance of fluorescence angiography to evaluate flow of blood vessels on the robotic system (Fig. 12.14). Indocyanine green is a helpful adjunct to guide additional release and resection if necessary. A 5 mg intravenous push is given, and fluorescence angiography appears within approximately 1 minute. A bilateral laparoscopic transversus abdominus plane (TAP) block is performed to aid in pain control during recovery. Various formulations can be used, depending on the institution. Some institutions use a mixture of 60 cc of 0.25% bupivacaine with epinephrine combined with 10 mg of decadron, while others use a mixture of 0.25% bupivacaine, 1% lidocaine, and injectable saline, for example.

If lymphatic drainage is recognized after dissection intraoperatively, control can be obtained with clips or suture ligation to avoid lymphatic ascites. Following assessment of the lymphadenectomy and ganglionectomy bed for hemostasis and lymphatic leak, the liver retractor is removed, the robot undocked, and port sites closed in the usual fashion. The procedure is typically well tolerated, with most patients discharging from the hospital on postoperative day 1.

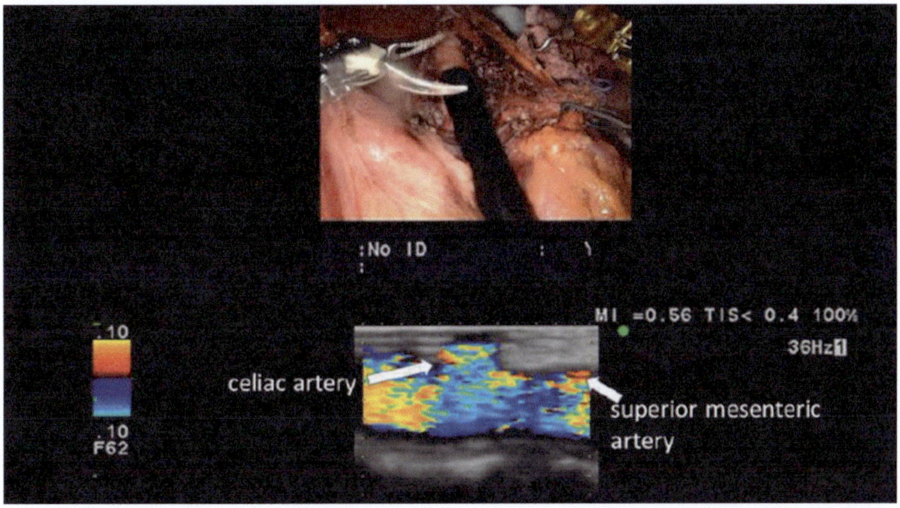

Fig. 12.13 Post-release ultrasound confirming no median arcuate ligament compression and improved diameter and blood flow through the celiac artery

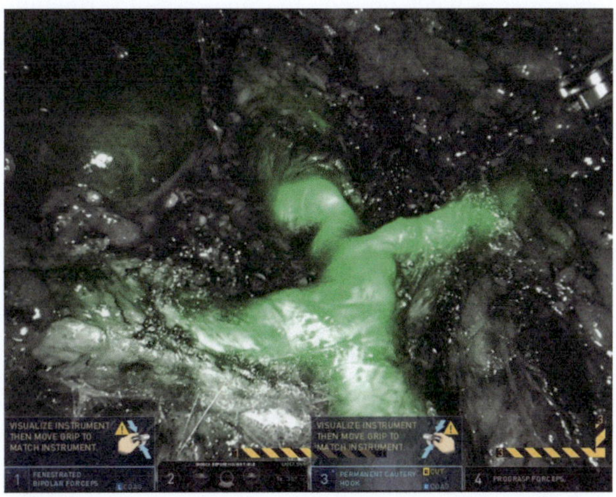

Fig. 12.14 Indocyanine green fluorescence angiography demonstrating blood flow through the celiac artery and its tributaries

Common Pitfalls and Anatomic Variants

With robotic surgery, there are unique challenges given the concern for conversion and separation from the patient while operating at the robot console. Great consideration needs to be taken regarding the potential for conversion with plans in place for how to convert, rapidly undock the robot, and control bleeding if necessary. When a surgeon is first starting to perform robotic operations for MALS, the recommended setup includes an assistant port, liver retractor in the epigastrium, open retractor with blades attached, and a marked midline incision, so the team can convert rapidly (Fig. 12.2a) (see Sect. "Setup" at the beginning of this chapter for a detailed description of the setup). A two-surgeon approach is also preferable in the beginning; the bedside assistant should be an experienced surgeon who is well-prepared to handle a conversion. Additionally, vascular surgery should be immediately available. As experience with robotic MALS surgery increases, the need for adjunctive measures in the setup and experience of assistants may decrease.

When evaluating a patient with MALS, it is important to conduct a thorough review of the patient's preoperative computerized tomography angiography (CTA) scan, paying special attention to arterial and venous anatomy near the median arcuate ligament. Patients may have variations in the anatomy of their foregut vasculature, so these are identified, and technical adjustments planned before operating. During the operation, dissection is done carefully to account for variations not identified on imaging.

Inadvertent injury to the inferior phrenic artery, most commonly the right inferior phrenic artery, is a common reason for intraoperative bleeding. It is not uncommon for the phrenic arteries to be directly along the path of dissection. They can arise from the celiac artery cephalad to the left gastric artery takeoff or directly off the aorta caudal to the takeoff of the celiac trunk. Care should be taken to identify these arteries when present. In some cases, the right inferior phrenic artery and less commonly the left inferior phrenic artery must be ligated and sacrificed to allow for a safe dissection and complete release of the ligament (Fig. 12.15).

The left gastric vein may be close to the median arcuate ligament and celiac ganglion, often crossing over the celiac artery (Fig. 12.16). To facilitate complete release, this vein may need to be divided with clips as well. If present, addressing these vessels will likely be necessary before celiac ganglionectomy can be

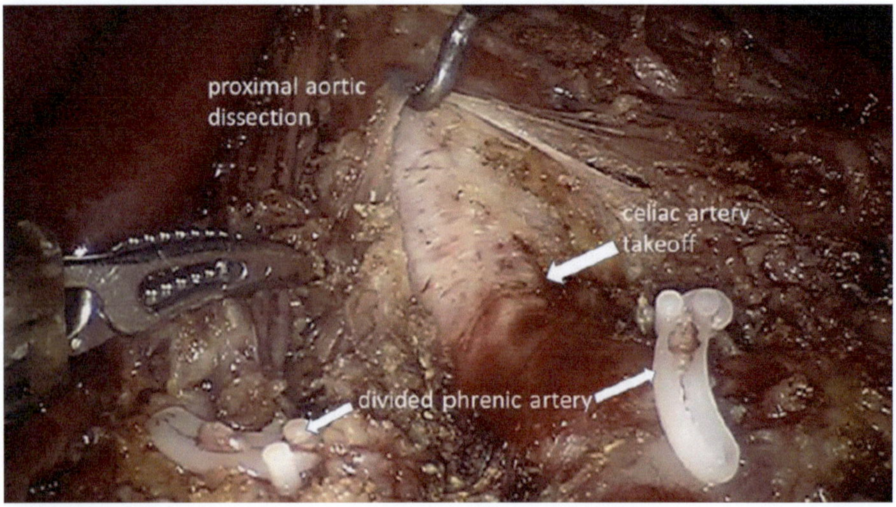

Fig. 12.15 Divided phrenic artery

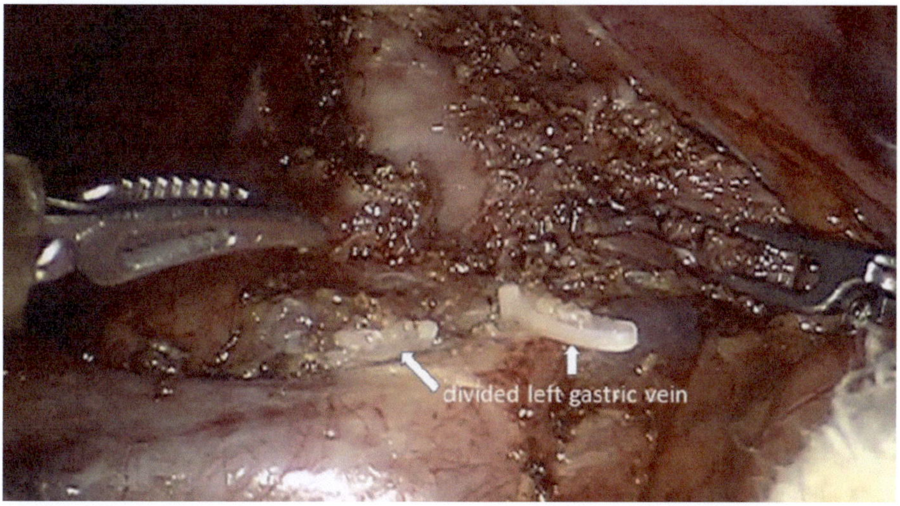

Fig. 12.16 Divided left gastric vein

completed. The left gastric vein is a tributary to the common hepatic vein. Care should be taken not to come across the left gastric vein during dissection and removal of the celiac ganglion and nerve plexus.

Significant lymphatic leakage often is a consequence of inadvertent injury to the cisterna chyli. This structure is often found near the intersection between the inferior vena cava and the common hepatic artery, medial to the main area of dissection. As such, one should avoid dissection that is too far medial to the median arcuate ligament and celiac trunk. As discussed above, if excessive leakage is noted intraoperatively, effort should be made to ligate the area of lymphatic drainage with a clip or suture.

Conclusions

Treating MALS robotically offers several potential advantages to aid the treating surgeon's technique and to ensure adequate release and resection, as well as to the patient's recovery. Surgery for MALS is performed within a confined space that is posterior to most intra-abdominal structures. Performing safe and meticulous surgery under such circumstances is where robotic surgery provides the most tangible benefit. The multiple degrees of articulation and steady camera provide a clear advantage over laparoscopic surgery in the setting of complex and high-risk surgery. With the increasing use of the robot, the publication of additional robotic series will be helpful to have a more robust library of evidence supporting its use and identify any pitfalls in its use that need troubleshooting. Resources and funding for hospitals to support the use of the robotic platform and training with proper robotic education are necessary to perform this operation optimally with successful outcomes. Minimally invasive laparoscopic or robotic MALS surgery is superior to open based on the available literature [4–6, 8, 10–13, 19, 20]. Minimally invasive surgical techniques are thought to demonstrate better pain outcomes and more reproducible technique [3, 7], although further studies are needed to support these claims.

References

1. El-Hayek KM, Titus J, Bui A, Mastracci T, Kroh M. Laparoscopic median arcuate ligament release: are we improving symptoms? J Am Coll Surg. 2013;216:272–9. https://doi.org/10.1016/j.jamcollsurg.2012.10.004.
2. Okamura AM. Haptic feedback in robot-assisted minimally invasive surgery. Curr Opin Urol. 2009;19(1):102. https://doi.org/10.1097/MOU.0B013E32831A478C.
3. Romero-Velez G, Barajas-Gamboa JS, Pantoja JP, et al. A nationwide analysis of median arcuate ligament release between 2010 and 2020: a NSQIP study. Surg Endosc. 2022;37:140–7. https://doi.org/10.1007/s00464-022-09431-3.
4. Fernstrum C, Pryor M, Wright GP, Wolf AM. Robotic surgery for median arcuate ligament syndrome. JSLS: Journal of the Society of Laparoscopic & Robotic Surgeons. 2020;24(2):1–7. https://doi.org/10.4293/JSLS.2020.00014.
5. Thoolen SJJ, Van Der Vliet WJ, Kent TS, et al. Technique and outcomes of robot-assisted median arcuate ligament release for celiac artery compression syndrome. J Vasc Surg. 2015;61(5):1278–84. https://doi.org/10.1016/j.jvs.2014.10.084.
6. Gerull WD, Sherrill W, Awad MM. Robotic median arcuate ligament release: management algorithm and clinical outcomes from a large minimally invasive series. Surg Endosc. 2022;1:1–7. https://doi.org/10.1007/S00464-022-09545-8/TABLES/3.
7. DeCicco J, Raja F, Ganesan S, El-Hayek K. First description of a histopathologic grading system and relationship to outcomes after robotic median arcuate ligament release with celiac ganglionectomy and lymphadenectomy. Surgery. 2024;175(3):822–32. https://doi.org/10.1016/J.SURG.2023.09.024.
8. Shin TH, Rosinski B, Strong A, et al. Robotic versus laparoscopic median arcuate ligament (MAL) release: a retrospective comparative study. Surg Endosc. 2022;36(7):5416–23. https://doi.org/10.1007/S00464-021-08877-1/TABLES/4.
9. Dunbar JD, Molnar W, Beman FF, Marable SA. Compression of the celiac trunk and abdominal angina. Am J Roentgenol Radium Therapy, Nucl Med. 1965;95(3):731–44. https://doi.org/10.2214/AJR.95.3.731.
10. Khrucharoen U, Juo YY, Chen Y, Jimenez JC, Dutson EP. Short- and intermediate-term clinical outcome comparison between laparoscopic and robotic-assisted median arcuate ligament release. J Robot Surg. 2020;14(1):123–9. https://doi.org/10.1007/S11701-019-00945-Y/TABLES/3.
11. Magnus L, Chakfé N, Lejay A, Thaveau F. Robot assisted laparoscopy for median arcuate ligament syndrome relief. EJVES Vasc Forum. 2022;56:32–6. https://doi.org/10.1016/J.EJVSVF.2022.06.002.
12. Do MV, Smith TA, Bazan HA, Sternbergh WC, Abbas AE, Richardson WS. Laparoscopic versus robot-assisted surgery for median arcuate ligament syndrome. Surg Endosc. 2013;27(11):4060–6. https://doi.org/10.1007/S00464-013-3061-X/TABLES/4.
13. Podda M, Pietro GG, Balestra F, et al. Robotic-assisted approach to median arcuate ligament syndrome with left gastric artery originating directly from the aorta. Report of a case and review of the current mini-invasive treatment modalities. Int J Med Robot Comp Assist Surg. 2018;14(4):e1919. https://doi.org/10.1002/RCS.1919.

14. Bustos R, Papamichail M, Mangano A, Valle V, Giulianotti PC. Robotic approach to treat median arcuate ligament syndrome: a case report. J Surg Case Rep. 2020;2020(5):1–4. https://doi.org/10.1093/JSCR/RJAA088.
15. You JS, Cooper M, Nishida S, Matsuda E, Murariu D. Treatment of median arcuate ligament syndrome via traditional and robotic techniques. Hawaii J Med Public Health. 2013;72(8):279–81.
16. Meyer M, Gharagozloo F, Nguyen D, Tempesta B, Strother E, Margolis M. Robotic-assisted treatment of celiac artery compression syndrome: report of a case and review of the literature. Int J Med Robot Comput Assist Surg. 2012;8(4):379–83. https://doi.org/10.1002/RCS.1448.
17. Relles D, Moudgill N, Rao A, Rosato F, Dimuzio P, Eisenberg J. Robotic-assisted median arcuate ligament release. J Vasc Surg. 2012;56(2):500–3. https://doi.org/10.1016/J.JVS.2012.02.057.
18. Jaik NP, Stawicki SP, Weger NS, Lukaszczyk JJ. Celiac artery compression syndrome: successful utilization of robotic-assisted laparoscopic approach. J Gastrointestin Liver Dis. 2007;16(1):93–6.
19. Roayaie S, Jossart G, Gitlitz D, Lamparello P, Hollier L, Gagner M. Laparoscopic release of celiac artery compression syndrome facilitated by laparoscopic ultrasound scanning to confirm restoration of flow. J Vasc Surg. 2000;32(4):814–7. https://doi.org/10.1067/MVA.2000.107574.
20. El-Hayek K. Robotic median arcuate ligament release. Atlas of Robotic Upper Gastrointestinal Surgery. 2022:1–8. https://doi.org/10.1007/978-3-030-86578-8_1 Published online.

Chapter 13
Perioperative Anesthesia Considerations for Median Arcuate Ligament Syndrome

Michael Platten, Maninder Singh, Vipul Dhumak, Nicolas M. Mas D. Alessandro, and Luis Tollinche

Introduction

Median arcuate ligament syndrome (MALS), also known as celiac artery compression syndrome, presents unique challenges in anesthesia management due to its complex etiology and varied symptomatology. Anesthesia considerations for patients with MALS focus on optimizing perioperative care to minimize the risk of exacerbating ischemia and associated complications. Preoperative evaluation should include a thorough assessment of symptoms, nutritional status, and comorbidities. It is crucial to ensure adequate preoperative fasting to reduce the risk of postprandial symptoms during the perioperative period [1]. During anesthesia induction, careful attention should be paid to hemodynamic stability, as these patients may be at increased risk of hemodynamic instability due to underlying vascular compromise. Maintenance of adequate perfusion pressure is essential to prevent further ischemia. Intraoperatively, maintaining normovolemia and avoiding hypotension are paramount. Postoperatively, close monitoring in a high-dependency or intensive care setting may be necessary, especially in patients with significant symptoms or comorbidities. Early mobilization and initiation of enteral nutrition should be considered to optimize recovery.

General anesthesia with endotracheal intubation and muscle relaxation is the choice of anesthesia used for surgery for correction of MALS, especially for the laparoscopic approach. Regional anesthesia is also used for intraoperative and postoperative pain control for open procedures. With the minimally invasive approach, an epidural catheter is not usually needed. Transversus abdominis plane (TAP)

M. Platten · M. Singh · V. Dhumak · N. M. M. D. Alessandro · L. Tollinche (✉)
Department of Anesthesiology and Pain Management, The MetroHealth System,
Case Western Reserve University School of Medicine, Cleveland, OH, USA
e-mail: mplatten@osteo.wvsom.edu; msingh@metrohealth.org; vdhumak1@metrohealth.org; nmasdalessandro@metrohealth.org; ltollinche@metrohealth.org

D. Shouhed et al. (eds.), *Median Arcuate Ligament Syndrome*,
https://doi.org/10.1007/978-3-031-80740-4_13

block, rectus sheath block, and local infiltration are generally used for these approaches [2]. Analgesic requirement can be very high during surgical manipulation of the median arcuate ligament and the celiac trunk [1]. There is a risk of injury to vital organs and important vascular structures during the surgery. The anesthesiologist needs to adapt to intraoperative physiological changes and the potential risk of complications due to injury. The combination of these considerations can make MALS surgery challenging for the anesthesiologist [1]. The choice of anesthesia, analgesia, monitoring, and attention to hemodynamic changes and possible complications are extremely important to prevent any anesthetic complications.

POTS, EDS, gastroparesis, GERD, and mast cell activation syndrome (MCAS) are commonly associated conditions with MALS, which are of anesthetic significance. These concomitant illnesses present MALS patients with unique anesthetic considerations in preoperative, intraoperative, and postoperative phases as POTS, EDS, MCAS, and gastroparesis have their own special anesthetic considerations and need to be managed carefully.

Perioperative Evaluation and Workup

The preoperative anesthesia evaluation is indispensable to optimize the chances of a successful anesthetic administration and surgical intervention. The perioperative workup for a patient with MALS starts with a thorough discussion with the patient about their past medical and surgical histories, comorbidities, and concerns going into surgery. The anesthesiologist will then have the necessary information to complete a physical exam, ensuring to address all critical body systems and patient-specific comorbidities before a plan of care is established.

MALS is a unique condition and has been seen to be present in various patient populations. Research has shown that the greatest prevalence of patients diagnosed with MALS and undergoing surgery for decompression are females with a thin body composition between the ages of 30 and 50 [3]. The ratio of females to males in MALS diagnoses is 4:1 [3]. There have also been cases seen within the pediatric population that have required surgical intervention [4]. Due to the variability within the patient population, the comorbidities that patients present with can be diverse. It is highly important for the preoperative assessment of the patient to mitigate modifiable risk factors prior to the induction of anesthesia to allow for optimized intraoperative management and favorable surgical outcome [5]. Studies have found that patients diagnosed with MALS, including pediatric patients, who also have psychiatric comorbidities may have impaired post-surgical outcomes and quality of life after recovery [6, 7]. Examples of these comorbid psychiatric conditions are post-traumatic stress disorder (PTSD), substance abuse, anxiety, and depression [8]. A psychological consult preoperatively may benefit the patient as to educate the patient in coping with their surgery while optimizing their chances of a successful surgery and recovery process [7, 9].

MALS symptoms often coincide with other gastroenterological disease symptoms, such as postprandial pain, nausea, vomiting, weight loss, diarrhea, and fatigue [10]. Therefore, a MALS diagnosis is often reached by exclusion, as it is secondary to other more acute gastroenterological pathology [1]. One case series found the average duration of symptoms prior to diagnosis was 34 months [11]. Thus, many of the patients undergoing surgery for MALS have had an extensive amount of testing and imaging done prior to their surgery. Examples of the pre-MALS diagnosis imaging and testing may include a complete upper gastrointestinal series, oral cholecystography, barium enema, intravenous urography, endoscopy, abdominal CT scan, and colored Doppler ultrasound of the celiac artery, HIDA scan, magnetic resonance angiography, more [1, 12]. Other adjunctive modalities include gastric exercise tonometry and celiac ganglion block [2]. Patients with MALS have often not obtained the pain relief they are looking for from the various prior interventions. Therefore, patients with MALS may be using opioids, alcohol, marijuana, or other drugs to self-medicate for temporary relief [8]. It is imperative for the anesthesia team to review the patient's test results preoperatively to gain a full understanding of the patient and their history prior to induction.

As much of the gastrointestinal preoperative testing has already been completed, in many instances, the anesthesiologist will not need to order further GI testing but rather review the results of the studies and order any anesthesia or procedure-specific testing to properly evaluate the patient's comorbidities. These procedure-specific tests ordered by the anesthesiologist will often evaluate the cardiac, pulmonary, and renal functions of the patient. For patients with cardiac comorbidities, the anesthesia team may recommend a preoperative electrocardiogram (ECG), echocardiogram, or cardiac stress test. They can evaluate the cardiac function of the patient using the Revised Cardiac Risk Index (RCRI) to help predict any cardiac complications prior to surgery [13]. To address any pulmonary concerns, the anesthesiologist may order a pulmonary function test (PFT) or pulmonology consult prior to induction. Lastly, renal function may be evaluated via a preoperative blood panel. All of the information gained from the preoperative testing will allow for the anesthesia team to properly categorize the patient's operative risk on a scale of 1–5, which has been shown to have significant ties to predict morbidity and mortality in patients undergoing any surgical procedure [14].

Medication management is essential in the treatment of patients with MALS preoperatively. The patient and their family members, especially in the case of pediatric patients with MALS, must be educated on the proper medications to take and to stop prior to surgery. To make appropriate recommendations, the anesthesia team should take a thorough medication and drug use history. The discussion of their medication and drug history will ensure the patient's suitability for surgery, mitigate the risks of intraoperative complications, allow for the proper dosing of anesthesia and analgesia, and optimize the probability of a successful anesthetic process and surgical recovery.

The use of enhanced recovery protocols (ERP) for all operations has become a novel way to increase the level of care for patients while improving surgical outcomes [15]. There are various key elements included in the ERP protocols including preoperative counseling, nutrition optimization, standardized anesthetic approaches, and early postoperative mobilization [15].

Through a complete preoperative evaluation and physical exam, the patient's history, comorbidities, and concerns can be addressed prior to induction and the start of surgery. These comorbidities may be physical or psychological and should be addressed to optimize the success of the surgical intervention and recovery process. After reviewing the preoperative test results and ordering any procedure-specific testing necessary for the patient, the anesthesia team will be equipped with the knowledge to implement the ERP protocols to optimize the patient for the successful surgical decompression of the median arcuate ligament.

Anesthesia and Disease Interaction

Patients with MALS present with unique anesthetic concerns. This patient population requires meticulous preoperative, intraoperative, and postoperative attention to ensure their health and safety during the procedure. MALS is a distinctive diagnosis, and it is often accompanied by various concomitant illnesses. The presentation of EDS, gastroparesis, GERD, and POTS is variable within patients with MALS, and each condition must be addressed individually to ensure the safety and efficacy of the patient during anesthesia.

EDS is a group of hereditary connective tissue disorders that are characterized by various clinical presentations, such as skin hyperextensibility, hypermobility of joints, fragility of blood vessels, and more [16]. Thirteen variants of EDS have been identified and are currently classified according to their genome [16]. The variant of EDS should be identified preoperatively as each has its own clinical manifestations [17]. There are numerous anesthetic concerns of patients with MALS with EDS starting with the minimal spread of local anesthetic through the fascia and thus leading to higher local anesthetic doses needed. Patient positioning is also crucial as patients with concomitant EDS have hypermobility of their joints and are thus prone to subluxations and must be kept in an anatomical position [18]. When inducing anesthesia and intubating the patient, providers must use caution as the craniocervical instability in EDS patients may lead to difficult intubations [18]. Additionally, EDS patients have an increased tissue fragility, which may cause issues during intubation [17]. Any instrumentation used during the intubation must be used with caution as the patient may have an increased susceptibility to bleeding, which could lead to a compromised airway [17]. Thus, video laryngoscopy should be considered during the induction and intubation of a patient with MALS with concomitant EDS.

During surgery, the management of a patient with MALS and concomitant EDS must be supervised extensively for numerous reasons. The first is that laparoscopic surgery might result in a higher inspiratory pressure to achieve normocapnia during peritoneal inflation. Hypercapnia will lead to acidosis and interfere with normal physiologic functions. Increased inspiratory pressures will lead to increased intrathoracic pressures, leading to decreased venous return and hemodynamic instability.

Secondly, there is an increased risk of pneumothorax due to spontaneous bullae rupture. Finally, due to the increased tissue fragility, bowel injury may occur after trivial trauma to the bowel. The anesthesia and surgery teams must be cognizant of this and be ready to properly manage the patient if complications due to the patient's respiratory status or tissue fragility arise.

Patients with MALS require intricate monitoring during surgery. Thus, various forms of monitoring are used. In most patients, standard ASA monitors including EKG, pulse oximetry, ETCO2, noninvasive blood pressure monitoring and temperature are adequate. Based on comorbidities, some patients may require additional invasive monitoring like an arterial line to monitor changes in blood pressure, fluid shifts, and cardiac output.

POTS is characterized by orthostatic intolerance associated with orthostatic tachycardia without orthostatic hypotension [19]. This is an autonomic system failure that gives rise to an increased risk of hemodynamic instability and collapse [19]. Preoperatively, a fluid bolus is recommended to minimize any hemodynamic changes associated with hypovolemia. Intraoperatively, there are many points and concerns to address. With a patient who has POTS, the anesthesia team should avoid sympathomimetic drugs and tachycardic inducing agents, such as ephedrine, glycopyrrolate, and epinephrine if possible. The avoidance of these medications will help maintain cardiac rate stability in the patient by not exposing them to tachycardic agents unnecessarily. Phenylephrine should be the vasopressor of choice to maintain adequate blood pressure levels without inducing tachycardia in a patient with POTS [20]. During the case, the anesthesia team aims to prevent precipitating events like inadequate anesthesia. Simultaneously, the team should aim to provide adequate pain relief and continue to maintain a tolerable level of pain postoperatively. Patients with MALS who present with concomitant POTS need to be anesthetically managed very closely throughout the entire perioperative period to prevent complications.

GERD is an exceptionally significant diagnosis in terms of anesthetic management as this condition is highly prevalent in the general population and the risks of anesthesia are increased. The primary risk of patients with GERD is pulmonary aspiration. With protective airway reflexes being impaired due to anesthesia, a patient with GERD is much more likely to regurgitate stomach contents into the esophagus which is extremely dangerous and can be a fatal anesthetic complication. Pulmonary aspiration is a highly serious anesthetic complication as it can bring lethal consequences after injury to the lungs from stomach matter, acid, and bacteria [21]. To optimize the anesthetic and surgical processes, the patient must properly follow all NPO guidelines. The patient should also be given antacids, an H2 antagonist, or a proton pump inhibitor (PPI) prophylactically before induction of anesthesia. In some cases, an orogastric (OG) or nasogastric (NG) tube may be placed to empty all stomach contents. This will help ensure the stomach is empty prior to the patient undergoing anesthesia and will minimize the risk of pulmonary aspiration during the case.

Gastroparesis is a condition marked by delayed gastric emptying. Just as with GERD, the primary risk of anesthesia for patients with MALS with gastroparesis is pulmonary aspiration. It is equally important for patients with gastroparesis to strictly adhere to NPO guidelines to optimize their chances of a successful anesthetic induction. Additionally, gastric point-of-care ultrasound (POCUS) is a novel method of analyzing the stomach contents prior to surgery [22, 23]. The performance of a point-of-care gastric ultrasound enables the anesthesia provider to assess patients at an increased risk for aspiration [22]. A case series of 38 patients showed that after gastric POCUS was administered, 71% of patients had the timing or technique of their anesthesia altered as the results gave the anesthesia team newfound information about the patient [23]. An OG or NG tube may also be placed for gastric decompression to remove all stomach contents and minimize the risk of pulmonary aspiration during surgery. To prevent aspiration risk during induction, rapid sequence intubation may be indicated. There are many other possible diabetic complications such as microvascular disease and autonomic dysfunction in patients with gastroparesis [24].

Postoperative Care

After the operation is completed, patients are typically extubated in the operating room after they fulfill the criteria for extubation and are transported to the postanesthesia recovery unit (PACU). In the PACU, immediate concerns are nausea, vomiting, and pain. Pain is treated with a multimodal approach including NSAIDS, opioids, regional anesthesia techniques, and local infiltration. The minimally invasive approach generally leads to minimal pain medication and requirements for opioids. Postoperative epidural catheters can be performed for minimally invasive operations converted to an open approach. Postoperative nausea and vomiting (PONV) are prevented with a scopolamine (1.5 mg) transdermal patch and an aprepitant (10 mg) oral pill, given in the preoperative area. Ondansetron (4 mg) and dexamethasone (4 mg) can be given intraoperatively. Postoperative medications used for preventing PONV are Compazine (5–10 mg IV) and amisulpride (10 mg IV). Dexmedetomidine can be used for anxious and younger patients. Patients are admitted to the hospital for observation, and the typical length of stay is 1–2 days after minimally invasive surgery and 3–5 days after open surgery. Oral intake may be started within a few hours with the minimal invasive approach. Mortality and morbidity rates for these operations are very low. Pediatric patients undergoing surgery for MALS report 33% rate of recurrence or no improvement in symptoms [2]. ERP protocols can be followed to facilitate early recovery [2].

Infiltration of long-acting local anesthetic at the port site, extracting residual CO_2, and intraperitoneal subdiaphragmatic injection of local anesthetic are recommended to reduce opioid requirements [1]. Epidural anesthesia can speed up recovery and intravenous patient-controlled analgesia can also be used in patients without epidurals [1]. To assess the effectiveness of the corrective surgery, it is important to start oral intake. Adequate pain management is also important to assist with the restoration of normal gastrointestinal function [1].

ERP protocols are novel strategies to approach the perioperative care of surgical patients. A meta-analysis of various laparoscopic abdominal surgery studies has shown that ERP protocols combined with the laparoscopic approach for abdominal operations increased patients' recovery times and outcomes, without increasing readmission rates or perioperative mortality [25]. In colorectal surgery, ERP protocols are currently well -stablished as the best care [26].

ERP pathway effective for MALS surgery practiced at our institution are as follows:

1. **Preoperative Practices**.
   (a) Preoperative counseling and education.
      (i) To reduce anxiety and to prepare patients for the anticipated surgery and related events.
   (b) Preoperative fasting and preoperative carbohydrate load.
      (i) Preoperative fasting should not exceed 6 h for solids and 2 h for liquids. Carbohydrate loading is recommended the evening before and 2 h before induction of anesthesia.
   (c) Preanesthetic medication.
      (i) Avoidance of long-acting anxiolytic medications. Use of only short-acting medications in the preoperative area to reduce anxiety and for performing regional analgesia.
   (d) Antithrombotic prophylaxis.
      (i) LMWH or unfragmented heparin reduces the risk of thromboembolic events and should be started 2–12 h before the surgery. Intermittent pneumatic compression stocking should also be used.
2. **Perioperative Practices.**
   (a) Perioperative steroids.
      (ii) Dexamethasone 5–10 mg reduces intraoperative stress and PONV.
   (b) Antimicrobial prophylaxis and skin preparation.
      (iii) Single dose of intravenous antibiotic administered less than 1 h before skin incision. Skin preparation with chlorhexidine is better than the povidone-iodine solution.
   (c) Minimally invasive approach.
      (iv) Minimally invasive surgery is superior to an open approach for faster patient recovery, better pain control, and decreased length of stay.

(d) Preventing intraoperative hypothermia.

   (v) Perioperative normothermia should be maintained during MALS surgery. It reduces infection, blood loss, and perioperative morbidity. Active forced air warming techniques should be used.

3. **Postoperative Practices**.
   (a) Postoperative nutrition and early oral intake.

      (vi) Patients can eat as soon as bowel sounds return, and patients can tolerate oral intake. Regional/local analgesia with low-dose opioid use plays an important role.

   (b) Early mobilization.

      (vii) Early mobilization is encouraged from POD 1 until discharge. This reduces DVT and pulmonary complications.

   (c) Analgesia.

      (viii) Regional analgesia and local infiltration techniques can reduce opioid requirement and quicken recovery by aiding in early mobilization, early oral intake, and decrease in length of hospital stay.

   (d) Preventing postoperative nausea and vomiting (PONV).

      (ix) Multimodal approach using ondansetron (4 mg) and dexamethasone (4 mg) for PONV prophylaxis.

   (e) Fluid management.

      (x) Avoidance of hypervolemia, use of balanced crystalloids.

   (f) Postoperative glycemic control.

      (xi) Use sliding scale, subcutaneous insulin to maintain normoglycemia.

      (xii) IV dextrose/D50 and saline as well as patients may be at risk for hypoglycemia.

Conclusion

An in-depth perioperative evaluation and workup for MALS surgery is essential for the optimization of a successful surgery and recovery for the patient. With several concomitant illnesses such as GERD, gastroparesis, POTS, and EDS often coinciding with MALS, the anesthesia team must be extremely intricate in their perioperative workup and plan of care to ensure the safety of anesthesia for each patient. Novel ERP protocols help give the anesthesia team new approaches to perioperative care, thus helping to optimize the chances of a successful surgery and full recovery. With increased awareness of MALS, physicians can become quicker to diagnose

MALS in patients, intricately study the mechanism of MALS to fully understand the disease, and relieve patients of chronic gastroenterological symptoms to improve patient quality of life.

Conflicts of Interest All authors meet the Committee on Publication Ethics requirements for authorship. Disclosures include the following: Luis E. Tollinche (LET) is a grant recipient through Merck Investigator Studies Program (MISP) to fund clinical trials at MSKCC (NCT03808077). Luis E. Tollinche serves a consultancy and advisory role for Merck & Co. Pharmaceutical Company. Luis E. Tollinche serves a consultancy and advisory role for GE Healthcare. No other authors have any associated conflicts of interest to the best of our knowledge. No funding or financial support was received for this study.

Funding Statement This project was supported in part by the Clinical and Translational Science Collaborative (CTSC) of Cleveland, which is funded by the National Institutes of Health (NIH), National Center for Advancing Translational Science (NCATS), and Clinical and Translational Science Award (CTSA) grant, UL1TR002548. The content is solely the responsibility of the authors and does not necessarily represent the official views of the NIH.

References

1. Álvarez-Fuente E, Fadrique Fuentes A, Poves-Álvarez R, Gómez-Pesquera E, Hernández LA. Anaesthetic management of median arcuate ligament syndrome. Rev Esp Anestesiol Reanim (Engl Ed). 2018;65(10):597–600. https://doi.org/10.1016/j.redar.2018.06.004. English, Spanish. Epub 2018 Jul 23
2. Vuong DT, Moak JP, Verghese ST, et al. Median arcuate ligament release in patients with POTS. Anesth Manag Pediatr Gen Surg. 2021:203–12. https://doi.org/10.1007/978-3-030-72551-8_14.
3. Kim EN, Lamb K, Relles D, Moudgill N, DiMuzio PJ, Eisenberg JA. Median arcuate ligament syndrome-review of this rare disease. JAMA Surg. 2016;151(5):471–7. https://doi.org/10.1001/jamasurg.2016.0002.
4. Mak GZ, Lucchetti AR, Drossos T, Fitzsimmons-Craft EE, Accurso EC, Stiles-Shields C, Newman EA, Skelly CL. Pediatric chronic abdominal pain and median arcuate ligament syndrome: a review and psychosocial comparison. Pediatr Ann. 2016;45(7):e257–64. https://doi.org/10.3928/00904481-20160613-01.
5. Aronson S, Martin G, Gulur P, Lipkin ME, Lagoo-Deenadayalan SA, Mantyh CR, Attarian DE, Mathew JP, Kirk AD. Preoperative optimization: a continued call to action. Anesth Analg. 2020;130(4):808–10. https://doi.org/10.1213/ANE.0000000000004492.
6. Skelly CL, Stiles-Shields C, Mak GZ, Speaker CR, Lorenz J, Anitescu M, Dickerson DM, Boyd H, O'Brien S, Drossos T. The impact of psychiatric comorbidities on patient-reported surgical outcomes in adults treated for the median arcuate ligament syndrome. J Vasc Surg. 2018;68(5):1414–21., ISSN 0741-5214. https://doi.org/10.1016/j.jvs.2017.12.078.
7. Stiles-Shields C, Osos S, Heilbrun A, Feldman ECH, Mak GZ, Skelly CL, Drossos T. Targeting coping to improve surgical outcomes in pediatric patients with median arcuate ligament syndrome: feasibility study. Front Psychol. 2021;12:695435. https://doi.org/10.3389/fpsyg.2021.695435. PMID: 34744860; PMCID: PMC8569106
8. Lubell J. Managing MALS during surgery means addressing chronic pain." OR Manager, 21 June 2023, https://www.ormanager.com/managing-mals-during-surgery-means-addressing-chronic-pain/.

9. Stiles-Shields C, Skelly CL, Mak GZ, Speaker C, Boyd H, O'Brien S, Drossos T. Psychological factors and outcomes in the surgical treatment of pediatric patients with median arcuate ligament syndrome. J Pediatr Gastroenterol Nutr. 2018;66(6):866–71. https://doi.org/10.1097/MPG.0000000000001900.
10. Okobi OE, Afuda BA, Boms M, Ekpemiro CU, Umeh NJ, Nnaji CG, Onyechi NP, Faderin OG, Chiji-Aguma JC, Stephen E, Amadi CO. Median arcuate ligament syndrome: management and literature review. Cureus. 2022;14(9):e28889. https://doi.org/10.7759/cureus.28889. PMID: 36225522; PMCID: PMC9542491
11. Sultan S, Hynes N, Elsafty N, Tawfick W. Eight years experience in the management of median arcuate ligament syndrome by decompression, celiac ganglion sympathectomy, and selective revascularization. Vasc Endovasc Surg. 2013;47(8):614–9. https://doi.org/10.1177/1538574413500536. Epub 2013 Aug 13
12. Reilly LM, Ammar AD, Stoney RJ, Ehrenfeld WK. Late results following operative repair for celiac artery compression syndrome. J Vasc Surg. 1985;2(1):79–91.
13. Davis C, Tait G, Carroll J, Wijeysundera DN, et al. The revised cardiac risk index in the new millennium: a single-centre prospective cohort re-evaluation of the original variables in 9,519 consecutive elective surgical patients. Can J Anaesth. 2013;60(9):855–63. https://doi.org/10.1007/s12630-013-9988-5. Epub 2013 Jun 28
14. Hackett NJ, De Oliveira GS, Jain UK, et al. ASA class is a reliable independent predictor of medical complications and mortality following surgery. Int J Surg. 2015;18:184–90. https://doi.org/10.1016/j.ijsu.2015.04.079. Epub 2015 Apr 30. PMID: 25937154
15. Melnyk M, Casey RG, Black P, Koupparis AJ. Enhanced recovery after surgery (ERAS) protocols: time to change practice? Can Urol Assoc J. 2011;5(5):342–8. https://doi.org/10.5489/cuaj.11002. PMID: 22031616; PMCID: PMC3202008
16. Miklovic T, Sieg VC. Ehlers-Danlos syndrome. 2023 may 29. In: StatPearls [internet]. Treasure Island, FL: StatPearls Publishing. p. 2023.
17. Johnston BA, Occhipinti KE, Baluch A, Kaye AD. Ehlers-Danlos syndrome: complications and solutions concerning anesthetic management. Middle East J Anaesthesiol. 2006;18(6):1171–84.
18. Chopra P, Bluestein L. Perioperative care in patients with Ehlers Danlos syndromes. Open J Anesthesiol. 2020;10:13–29. https://doi.org/10.4236/ojanes.2020.101002.
19. Grigoriou E, Boris JR, Dormans JP. Postural orthostatic tachycardia syndrome (POTS): association with Ehlers-Danlos syndrome and orthopaedic considerations. Clin Orthop Relat Res. 2015;473:722–8.
20. Rabbitts JA, Groenewald CB, Jacob AK, Low PA, Curry TB. Postural orthostatic tachycardia syndrome and general anesthesia: a series of 13 cases. J Clin Anesth. 2011;23(5):384–92. https://doi.org/10.1016/j.jclinane.2010.12.013. PMID: 21802629; PMCID: PMC3349351
21. Hayashi R, Maeda S, Hideki T, Higuchi H, Miyawaki T. Pulmonary aspiration during induction of general anesthesia. Anesth Prog. 2020;67(4):214–8. https://doi.org/10.2344/anpr-67-02-03. PMID: 33393603; PMCID: PMC7780261
22. Schwisow S, Falyar C, Silva S, Muckler VC. A protocol implementation to determine aspiration risk in patients with multiple risk factors for gastroparesis. J Perioper Pract. 2022;32(7–8):172–7. https://doi.org/10.1177/1750458921996925. Epub 2021 Jul 12
23. Alakkad H, Kruisselbrink R, Chin KJ, Niazi AU, Abbas S, Chan VW, Perlas A. Point-of-care ultrasound defines gastric content and changes the anesthetic management of elective surgical patients who have not followed fasting instructions: a prospective case series. Can J Anaesth. 2015;62(11):1188–95. https://doi.org/10.1007/s12630-015-0449-1. Epub 2015 Aug 4
24. Xiao MZX, Englesakis M, Perlas A. Gastric content and perioperative pulmonary aspiration in patients with diabetes mellitus: a scoping review. Br J Anaesth. 2021;127(2):224–35. https://doi.org/10.1016/j.bja.2021.04.008. Epub 2021 May 20

25. Li Z, Zhao Q, Bai B, Ji G, Liu Y. Enhanced recovery after surgery programs for laparoscopic abdominal surgery: a systematic review and meta-analysis. World J Surg. 2018;42(11):3463–73. https://doi.org/10.1007/s00268-018-4656-0.
26. Pędziwiatr M, Mavrikis J, Witowski J, Adamos A, Major P, Nowakowski M, Budzyński A. Current status of enhanced recovery after surgery (ERAS) protocol in gastrointestinal surgery. Med Oncol. 2018;35(6):95. https://doi.org/10.1007/s12032-018-1153-0. PMID: 29744679; PMCID: PMC5943369

Chapter 14
Arterial Considerations in Median Arcuate Ligament Syndrome

Woosup Michael Park and Jonathan C. Bartko

Introduction

The cause of the pain syndrome related to median arcuate ligament syndrome is controversial. There are those that propose regional mesenteric ischemia due to the celiac axis compression and have demonstrated changes in gastric mucosal perfusion in patients with MALS [1]. The contravening theory is that it is a nerve compression syndrome—the celiac plexus is compressed, resulting in injury and neuropathy with a pathologic pain response to stimuli [2]. There is data to support both concepts, but no evidence is sufficient for one to exclude the other. It may never be elucidated with clinical outcomes data as celiac plexus neurolysis likely plays a significant role in eliminating pain signals for both entities. The goal of MALS surgery is the release of the ligament-releasing celiac axis compression as well as neurolysis, and the metric for successful release, aside from relief of pain, is the reduction of celiac axis stenoses on follow-up duplex.

There is a model for this in another compression syndrome: thoracic outlet syndrome (TOS). TOS is categorized by what is compressed—arterial TOS (aTOS), venous TOS (vTOS), and neurogenic TOS (nTOS). aTOS and nTOS, while having different signs and symptoms, overlap because they share the space that is compressed in the thoracic outlet. Similarly, artery (celiac axis) and nerve (celiac plexus) share the compressed space under the median arcuate ligament. The authors propose a similar categorization of MALS into neurogenic MALS and arterial MALS.

Arterial MALS (aMALS) is arterial injury and disease caused by compression of the celiac axis by the median arcuate ligament marked by intimal injury, vessel remodeling, and periadventitial fibrosis. The diseases associated with aMALS are:

W. M. Park (✉) · J. C. Bartko
Harrington Heart and Vascular Institute, University Hospitals, Cleveland, OH, USA

Case Western Reserve University School of Medicine, Cleveland, OH, USA

D. Shouhed et al. (eds.), *Median Arcuate Ligament Syndrome*,
https://doi.org/10.1007/978-3-031-80740-4_14

1. Celiac axis aneurysm.
2. Celiac axis dissection.
3. Celiac axis stenosis or occlusion.
4. Visceral artery aneurysm.
5. Foregut mesenteric ischemia.
6. Celiac axis inflammation and fibrosis with intimal injury.

Anatomy

The abdominal viscera are divided into the foregut (the stomach, duodenum, liver, pancreas, and spleen), midgut (the small intestines and right colon), and hindgut (the transverse colon through rectum). The celiac axis supplies the foregut, the superior mesenteric artery the midgut, and the IMA and hypogastric branches the hindgut. There are important collaterals between the three visceral arteries as well as anatomic variations, which are important to be aware of in managing patients with aMALS, as the celiac axis is compressed and frequently injured from long-term compression [3].

The median arcuate ligament is the latching point of the posterior diaphragm to the spine (Fig. 14.1). This develops after the descent of the diaphragm from the neck, pushed down by the growing lungs, and after the development of the celiac axis. In up to 5% of patients undergoing CT scanning of the abdomen at an academic center,

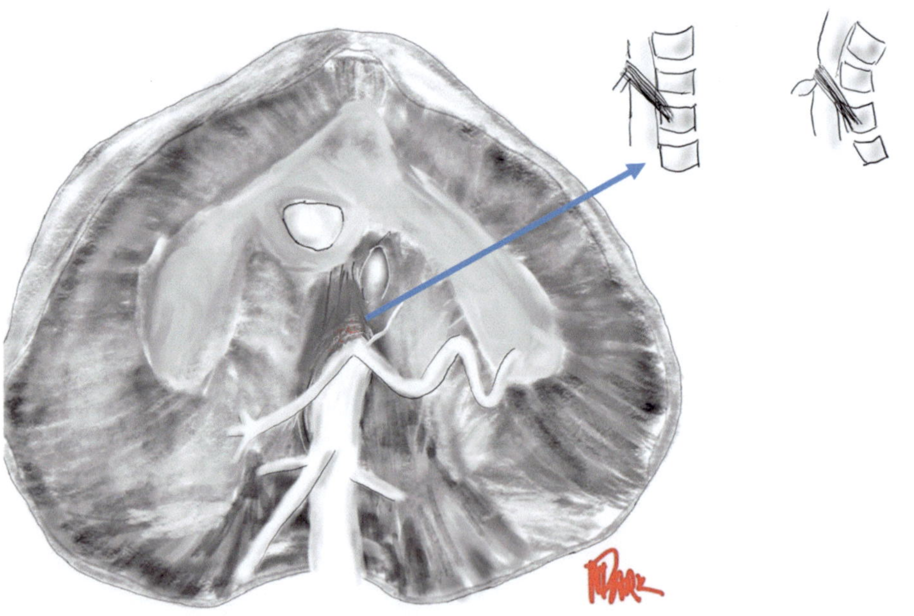

Fig. 14.1 Pathoanatomy of the median arcuate ligament

the median arcuate ligament compresses the origin of the celiac axis [4]. Respiration, posture, and spinal curvature contribute to the compression. A hemodynamically significant compression will result in respirophasic velocity elevation on duplex ultrasound: elevated on expiration, normalized on inspiration. On a CTA, depending on the phase of respiration during the breath hold, there may be a hook sign. There may be a kink or stenosis, post-stenotic dilatation, dissection, occlusion, or aneurysm of the celiac axis.

The left gastric artery branches first from the celiac axis (Fig. 14.2), one of several arteries feeding the stomach. The celiac axis continues for another 2–3 cm before dividing into the splenic and common hepatic arteries.

The common hepatic artery courses on and gives off the gastroduodenal artery and continues as the proper hepatic before dividing into the right and left hepatic arteries. There are important variations, including a common celiomesenteric trunk, replaced right or left hepatic artery with origination from the superior mesenteric artery, celiac axis, or aorta.

The collateral circulation between the celiac axis and superior mesenteric artery has been typically described as robust, but this is from the experience of atherosclerotic mesenteric arterial occlusive disease where collaterals develop over time and is potentially not the case with an acute event. Also, in trauma and aneurysm repair, the celiac axis is sometimes intentionally occluded as part of therapy with the understanding that the collateral supply is sufficient from the superior mesenteric artery. The key point to understand is that in MALS, the acuity of occlusion onset and the combined compression of the celiac plexus must be considered in the workup. Aside from minor contribution from the spleen and gastroepiploic vessels, the most important collateral is the inferior pancreaticoduodenal artery (Fig. 14.2). This dominant collateral arises from the superior mesenteric artery and forms the Arc of Rio Branco via the inferior pancreaticoduodenal arcades to the

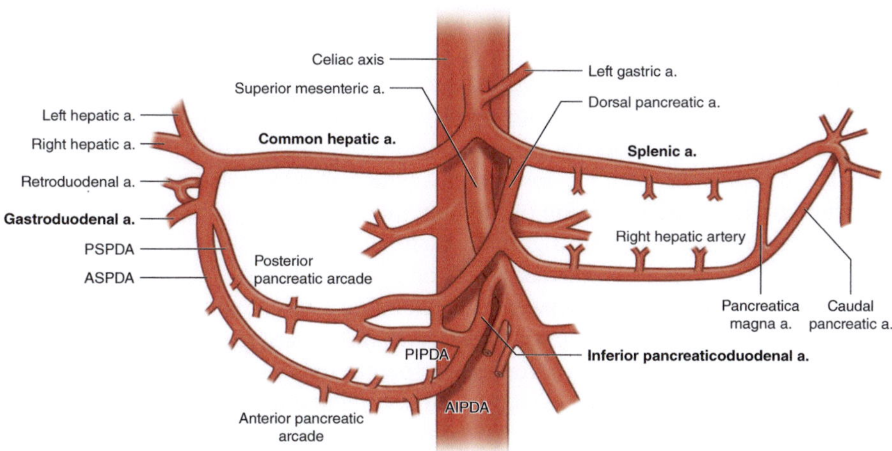

Fig. 14.2 Arterial anatomy of celiac axis

gastroduodenal artery and the Arc of Buhler via the inferior pancreaticoduodenal artery to the dorsal pancreatic artery. These collaterals can be visualized on CTA and contrast angiography through prominent filling, enlargement, and sometimes the presence of visceral aneurysms. In contrast, in angiography, collaterals flow in reversed direction, and in the instance of hemodynamically significant celiac axis compression, there is reversed flow in the gastroduodenal artery (Arc of Rio Branco) or the dorsal pancreatic artery (Arc of Buhler).

Atherosclerosis, arterial dissections, interventions, and surgical resections result in loss of these collaterals, and combined with celiac axis compression sets up a rare situation of foregut ischemia manifested as epigastric abdominal pain, pancreatitis, transaminitis, and ischemic ulcerations on endoscopy. These are late findings pain is usually the first and only symptom until these late findings occur. Pain by itself is nonspecific, and can result in diagnostic and treatment delay. Left untreated, these can potentially progress to organ death and mortality.

Case 1

The patient is a 41-year-old woman, without significant past medical history, who presented with severe back pain and who was found to have a 3 cm pancreaticoduodenal artery aneurysm and severe stenosis of the celiac axis due to median arcuate ligament compression. Arteriogram from the celiac axis showed a reversal of flow from the pancreaticoduodenal artery into the gastroduodenal artery. She underwent coil embolization of the pancreaticoduodenal artery aneurysm. Soon after discharge, she returned to the emergency department with severe epigastric abdominal pain. She reported the pain to be worse after eating. CTA and laboratory testing, including serum amylase, lipase, and liver function testing, were reported normal, and she was dismissed with analgesics and antacids. The patient lost 12 pounds over the subsequent week and a half prior to consultation and on examination had severe epigastric pain and tenderness.

The patient was admitted for hydration and pain control. Laboratory testing was repeated and was normal, including white blood cell count, amylase, lipase, and liver function testing. Esophagogastroduodenoscopy was performed and was normal. The patient was taken for aortography, which showed patency of the superior mesenteric artery with occlusion of the large feeding collateral to the pancreaticoduodenal artery aneurysm. Aortography in lateral projection showed severe stenosis of the celiac axis by the median arcuate ligament (Fig. 14.3).

Her pain persisted. In the absence of hepatobiliary, pancreatic, and upper gastrointestinal pathology, or pain prior to visceral aneurysm embolization, the most likely diagnosis of her pain syndrome was foregut mesenteric ischemia. This was supported by the finding of severe limitation of foregut arterial supply by celiac axis compression and loss of collateral circulation due to the coiling of the pancreaticoduodenal artery aneurysm.

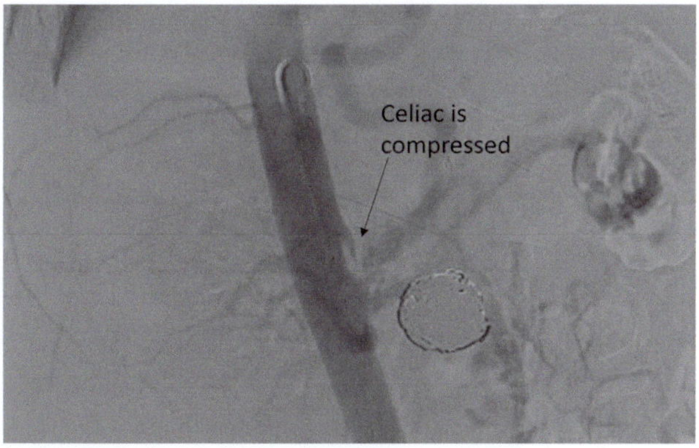

Fig. 14.3 Aortogram showing celiac axis compression

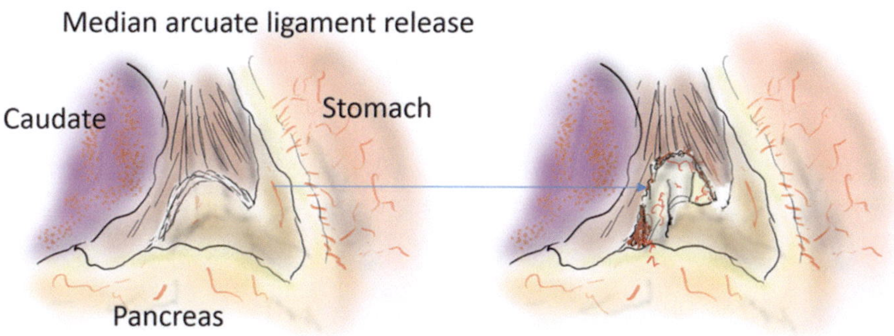

Fig. 14.4 Open median arcuate ligament release

The patient was taken to the operating room for laparotomy and open release of the celiac axis (Fig. 14.4). The artery was severely compressed, and the surrounding tissues were inflamed. Postoperatively, her diet was reintroduced and while she had incisional pain, the postprandial epigastric pain was gone. In follow-up, the patient had regained her lost weight and was recovering well.

Discussion

This patient developed chronic mesenteric ischemia of the foregut in the setting of celiac axis compression after losing her collateral from the superior mesenteric artery with treatment of a large pancreaticoduodenal artery aneurysm. Release of the median arcuate ligament and its compression on the celiac axis successfully resolved the patient's symptoms. The CTA obtained prior to the patient's aneurysm embolization shows a prominent collateral supplying the foregut (Fig. 14.5).

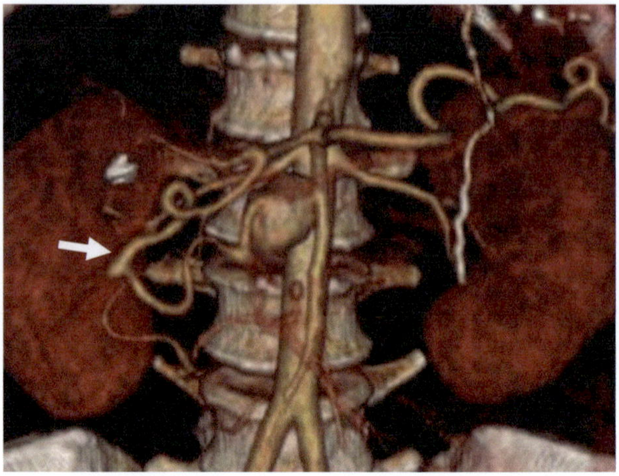

Fig. 14.5 CTA showing prominent collateral circulation (white arrow) due to celiac axis compression along with pancreaticoduodenal artery aneurysm

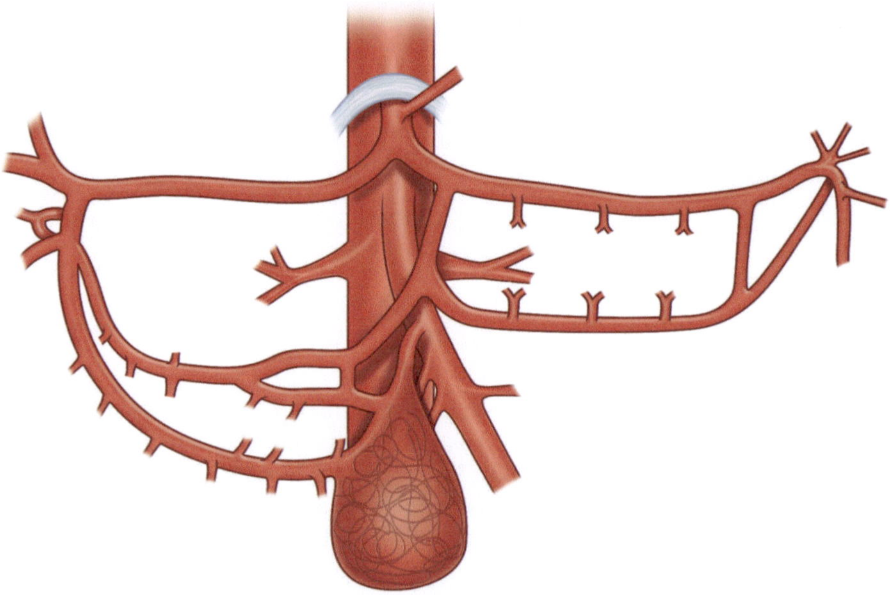

Fig. 14.6 Patient's celiac compression limited foregut perfusion after coiling of pancreaticoduodenal artery aneurysm

The patient did not have any pain prior to her presentation for the symptomatic pancreaticoduodenal artery aneurysm. The collateral suggested the circulation adjusted to the presence of the severe celiac axis compression. The association of visceral artery aneurysms in the pancreaticoduodenal and gastroduodenal arteries with median arcuate ligament compression is well-known [5].

In this patient, the compression was not associated with classic MALS, but the loss of the collateral brought on the symptoms associated with MALS: the postprandial epigastric abdominal pain and true foregut chronic mesenteric ischemia (Fig. 14.6). Similar phenomena are seen in patients with iliac artery occlusion who can be asymptomatic but develop claudication or rest pain with loss of collateral flow. Normal EGD is not unexpected as ischemic ulcerations, pancreatitis, and liver transaminitis are late, severe findings that are associated with morbidity and mortality. In this case, the patient had immediate relief, and this was sustained at several months of follow-up.

Arterial median arcuate ligament syndrome differs from the neurogenic median arcuate ligament syndrome in its association with visceral artery aneurysms and celiac artery aneurysms. The development of visceral aneurysms in the setting of celiac axis compression is not entirely clear but has been hypothesized to occur due to high volume, reversed flows in collateral arteries that are originally small such as in the hepatic, gastroduodenal, or pancreaticoduodenal arteries or their branches. Embolization of these aneurysms, which is the preferred treatment, often results in the loss of important collaterals while leaving behind a compressed celiac axis, which may limit the perfusion of an isolated bed. The most recent Society for Vascular Surgery (SVS) guidelines for visceral artery aneurysms recommend selective celiac revascularization in the setting of aneurysm treatment [6].

Case 2

The patient is a 68-year-old man with hypertension, hyperlipidemia, gout, and known hepatic artery aneurysm, who presented to the ED with sharp right upper quadrant abdominal pain. It hurt to breathe and he underwent a CT-PE, which ruled out a pulmonary embolism but showed growth of his common hepatic artery aneurysm from 20 to 24 mm in 2 years. He was admitted to the ICU for blood pressure control. With normotension, his abdominal pain remitted. On examination, his abdomen was soft, with an area of pain located in the right upper quadrant. His laboratory values were normal, including liver function testing. He had a CTA, which showed (Fig. 14.7) a 24 mm common hepatic artery (CHA) aneurysm with left and right hepatic arteries arising from the CHA, as well as a gastroduodenal artery. There was celiac axis compression by the median arcuate ligament and post-stenotic dilatation of the celiac axis to 13 mm.

Incidentally, there was an irregularity of the superior mesenteric artery, which was not iatrogenic from prior instrumentation. No other findings in the renal arteries or carotid arteries were present to suggest fibromuscular dysplasia (FMD).

The patient was brought to the operating room, and the CHA aneurysm as well as the aorta were exposed via a chevron incision. The celiac axis was fully exposed by releasing the median arcuate ligament. This area was affected by fibrotic tissue. The celiac axis visibly expanded upon the release of the ligament. The aneurysm was resected, and a bypass was performed from the normal hepatic artery to a patch

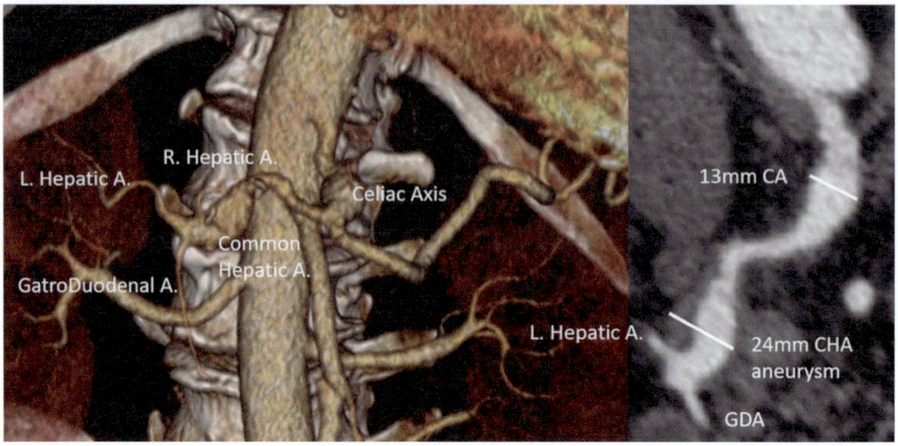

Fig. 14.7 Celiac axis compression with post-stenotic dilatation to 13 mm and a 24 mm common hepatic artery aneurysm

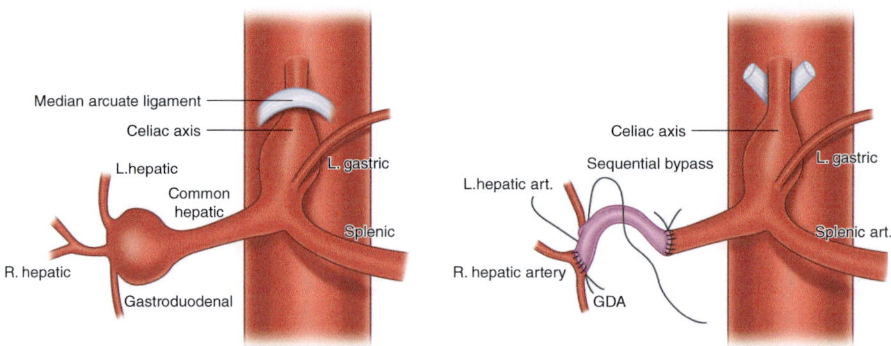

Fig. 14.8 Repair of common hepatic artery aneurysm with saphenous vein graft with preservation of visceral branches

incorporating the origins of the right hepatic and gastroduodenal arteries. A side-to-side anastomosis was performed to the right hepatic artery. The patient recovered uneventfully. In follow-up at 1 year, his bypass remained patent, and the celiac axis has not grown (Fig. 14.8).

Discussion

This case illustrates a common association between median arcuate ligament compression of the celiac axis and the presence of visceral artery aneurysms. In the current SVS guidelines [6], visceral artery aneurysms of the foregut (excluding splenic artery aneurysms) are recommended for repair at any size due to their propensity to rupture. The mechanism for this is not robustly supported by the data due to the rarity of these aneurysms. The presence of turbulent flow does play a role in the post-stenotic dilatation of the celiac axis, but it is uncertain how it can affect a downstream vessel. The closure of flow in the celiac axis and recruitment of collateral flow from the inferior pancreaticoduodenal artery as in Case#1 is conjectured to cause aneurysms because of high pressure reversed flow. The release of the median arcuate ligament eliminates the cause of the celiac axis dilatation and the source of turbulent flow. While this patient and the first were not tested for connective tissue disorders, there may be something about the substance of their arteries, which leaves them prone to visceral aneurysm development. This patient may have something akin to FMD involving the enlargement of his visceral arteries, but the final pathology made no mention of it.

While most visceral artery aneurysms can and should be treated with embolization, the location of this aneurysm precluded this, as perfusion of the liver would be lost. The use of saphenous vein graft confers durability but needs to be monitored for both patency and aneurysmal degeneration.

Regarding the repair of the celiac axis, a significant number of patients do have internal injuries to the intima (see Case 3) and should be considered for repair—typically with patch angioplasty, reimplantation, or bypass, if fixed stenosis is encountered during laparotomy, or with staged angioplasty and stent.

Case 3

The patient is a young woman in her twenties with complex symptoms of postprandial epigastric pain, left flank pain, and obstructive symptoms, who through extensive gastroenterological and vascular workup was found to have multiple compression syndromes, encompassing median arcuate ligament syndrome, superior mesenteric artery syndrome (SMAS), and nutcracker syndrome (NCS); who had undergone a laparoscopic median arcuate ligament release, a duodenojejunostomy for the SMAS, and a left kidney autotransplant for the NCS; and who had presented with recurrent symptoms of epigastric abdominal pain 2 years after her laparoscopic MAL release. There was some residual compression of the median arcuate ligament suggested by duplex and CTA, and she underwent redo-laparotomy and release of cicatricial tissues and remnant nerve fibers around the celiac axis. The celiac axis was fully released and after recovery from laparotomy, after which the patient had a brief symptom relief before the epigastric pain returned. Duplex showed a persistent velocity elevation in the celiac axis that was not respirophasic (Fig. 14.9).

The patient was taken for angiography and the celiac axis was stented. The patient had relief from her abdominal pain, which had lasted over a year at last followup visit. Testing at 1 year post-procedure shows a patent stent with improved velocity (Fig. 14.10).

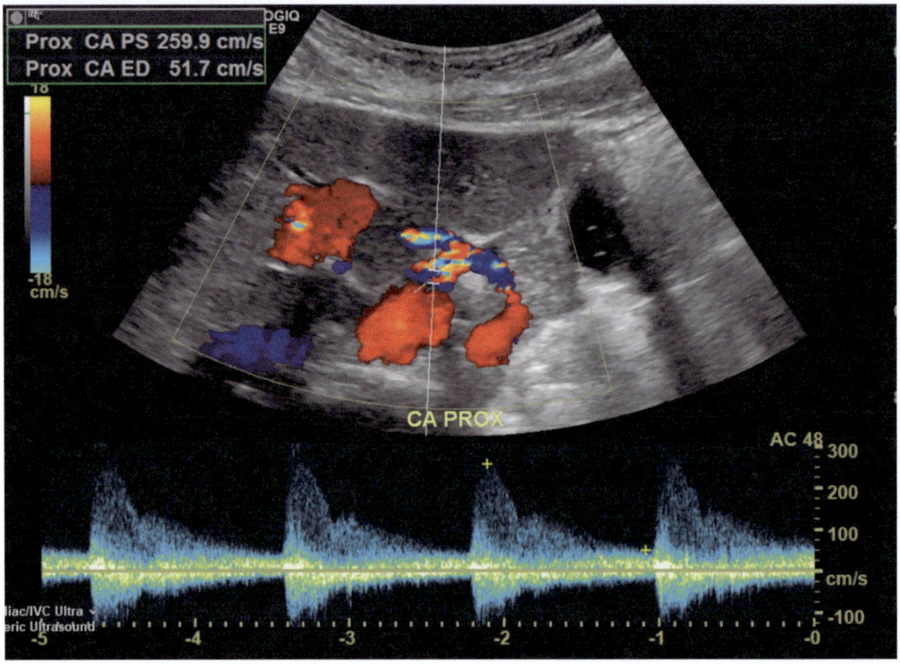

Fig. 14.9 Velocity elevations in celiac axis persisting after median arcuate ligament release suggest chronic intimal injury

Discussion

The patient with pain recurrence, after an initial period of relief, represents a significant minority of patients—up to 7–24% experience recurrence of pain [7, 8]. Imaging may show persistent or recurrent compression of the median arcuate ligament. Reoperation may reveal remnant ligament or plexus fibers. This pain may occur in the absence of a visible compression on the celiac axis. Pathology often reveals fibrosis as well as nerve tissue, and this may point to a pathoetiology, where remnant nerve endings develop neuromas within this scar tissue. The laparotomy was undertaken to remove as much overlying scar tissue as possible off the aorta and celiac axis. The persistence of pain then required a closer look at the artery.

In the past, when open surgery was the only option, median arcuate ligament release was often accompanied by celiac axis patch angioplasty. In many of these patients, external compression had resulted in intimal injury and hyperplasia. In a series from the 1980s, the University of California San Francisco (UCSF) group found that in patients who had celiac axis repair, typically in the form of patch angioplasty but also aorto-celiac or hepatic bypass, a higher percentage of patients had lasting relief compared to those who had release only [9]. In the era of robotic and laparoscopic median arcuate ligament release, there are two things that occur. The celiac axis is not repaired, and its revascularization is typically a staged

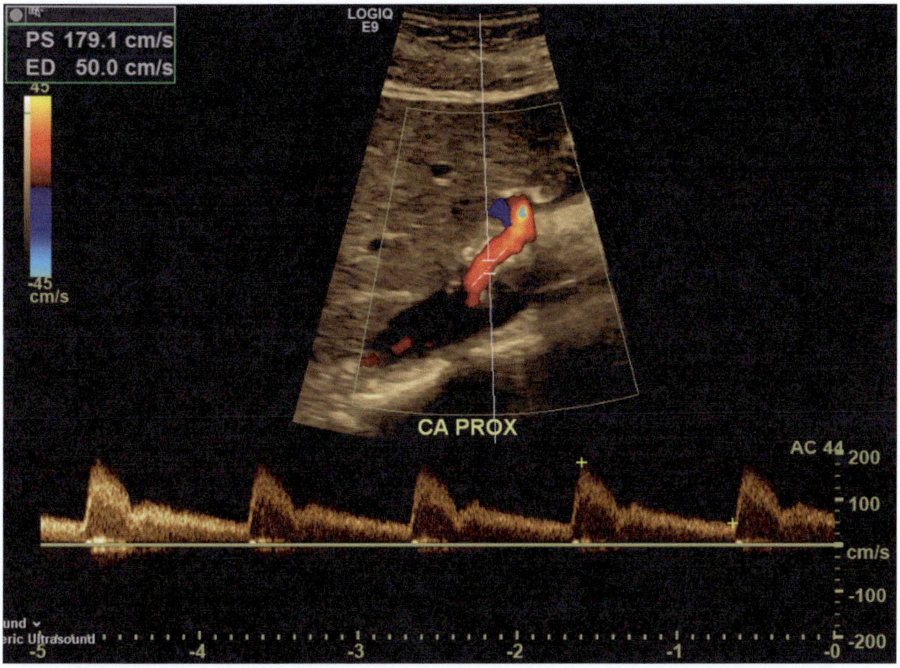

Fig. 14.10 Improved velocities after stent placement

angioplasty and stent if necessary—typically with patients who have persistent symptoms despite the release. The second issue is that laparoscopic and robotic releases have a steep learning curve and complete release is a challenge, particularly in light of the infrequent but morbid conversions that are needed for bleeding encountered during surgery. This last issue points out the Achilles' heel of minimally invasive surgery. Bailing out and repairing bleeding, which typically comes from the aorta or the celiac axis, requires vascular surgical skills, and being prepared to convert to open should be part of the routine setup in MALS operations.

In the setting of recurrent MALS pain or persistent MALS pain present 6 months after surgery, and with clearance of the median arcuate ligament and the finding of stenosis or occlusion on the mesenteric duplex, then revascularization— in the form of bypass, celiac axis patch angioplasty, or most commonly angioplasty and stenting—may offer relief from these symptoms.

Case 4

Patient is a 54-year-old man presenting with 3 years of chronic epigastric discomfort exacerbated by coughing and certain postures. The pain was made worse with eating, and he reported a 30-pound weight loss. Examination revealed epigastric

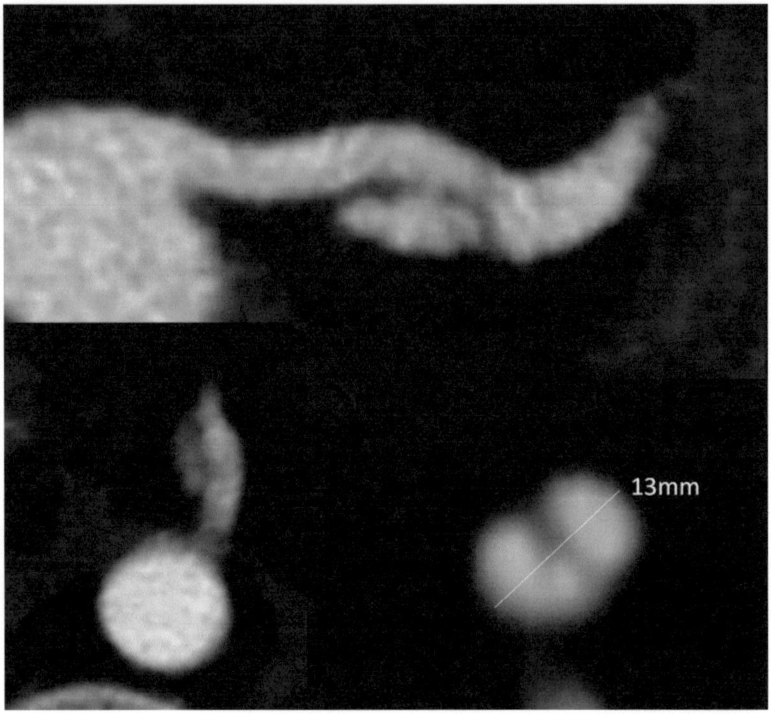

Fig. 14.11 CT scan centerline reconstruction shows dissection and aneurysmal degeneration in celiac axis secondary to celiac axis compression

abdominal pain and tenderness. There was an umbilical hernia. Duplex showed velocity elevations in the celiac axis consistent with stenosis over 70%. CTA showed a celiac axis compression with dissection and aneurysm of the celiac axis measuring 13 mm (Fig. 14.11).

He was sent for a celiac plexus block, and for the first time in years, he experienced relief from the epigastric abdominal pain. He was taken to the operating room for laparotomy for open release of the median arcuate ligament and aneurysmorraphy versus resection with bypass. Exploration revealed the aneurysm to start at the point where the ligament kinked the artery. The ligament was taken down, and the patient was heparinized after the celiac axis, aorta, and left gastric, common hepatic, and splenic arteries were controlled. The aneurysmal segment had good adventitia, offering the opportunity for primary closure. The aneurysm was opened, and the dissection flap resected (Fig. 14.12). A 12F shunt Argyle shunt was placed, and the aneurysm pared back and closed primarily over the shunt, which was directed from the aorta to the splenic artery. This allowed the celiac to be closed to an appropriate diameter without narrowing the artery. The patient recovered well and in follow-up had a widely patent celiac axis with complete relief of his abdominal pain symptoms.

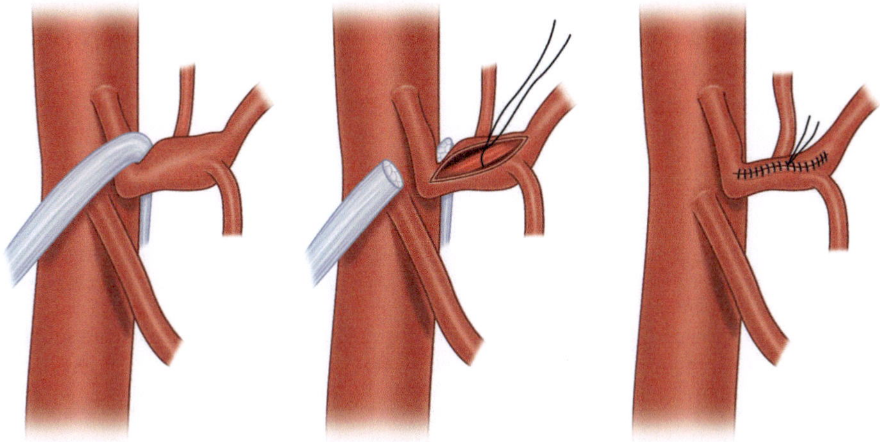

Fig. 14.12 Median arcuate ligament release and celiac aneurysmorrhaphy

Discussion

The median arcuate acts to compress the artery against the aorta for about 1–2 cm in most patients with MALS. Beyond this terminal edge of ligament, the artery flips upward and grinds against the edge of the ligament. This can result in intimal injury, dissection, and aneurysm formation as in this patient. It has even been reported multiple times in the literature that the celiac axis was avulsed after blunt trauma, which suggests that with sufficient force, the celiac axis can be scraped off the aorta by the median arcuate ligament [10, 11]. This case illustrates the role that the celiac plexus has in mediating pain from this area of injury. The epigastric pain, the post-prandial abdominal pain, and pain with breathing are all relieved by celiac plexus block and by surgical neurolysis. The arterial disease associated with it, the aMALS, necessarily had to be repaired via traditional open surgery. Hopefully, in the future, this repair can be done robotically or laparoscopically.

Conclusion

Arterial MALS cannot be separated from neurogenic MALS when it comes to pain and pain relief, but in specific circumstances, arterial considerations must be reviewed as part of the workup, including the endovascular and open surgical repairs of aneurysms, revascularization to address flow limiting lesions caused by chronic compression, and revascularization specifically to address loss of collateral flow in the setting of compression. As a final note, the observed phenomena of "acute MALS" that drives many patients to the emergency room, with occasional findings of pancreatitis or transaminitis, necessitates a careful review of the vascular anatomy to ensure adequate perfusion, understanding that endoscopic and laboratory findings are late, often irreversible findings in mesenteric ischemia.

References

1. Mensink PB, van Petersen AS, Kolkman JJ, Otte JA, Huisman AB, Geelkerken RH. Gastric exercise tonometry: the key investigation in patients with suspected celiac artery compression syndrome. J Vasc Surg. 2006;44:277–81.
2. Weber JM, Boules M, Fong K, Abraham B, Bena J, El-Hayek K, et al. Median arcuate ligament syndrome is not a vascular disease. Ann Vasc Surg. 2016;30:22–7.
3. Terlouw LG, Moelker A, Abrahamsen J, Acosta S, Bakker OJ, Baumgartner I, Boyer L, Corcos O, van Dijk LJ, Duran M, Geelkerken RH, Illuminati G, Jackson RW, Kärkkäinen JM, Kolkman JJ, Lönn L, Mazzei MA, Nuzzo A, Pecoraro F, Raupach J, Verhagen HJ, Zech CJ, van Noord D, Bruno MJ. European guidelines on chronic mesenteric ischaemia—joint United European Gastroenterology, European Association for Gastroenterology, Endoscopy and Nutrition, European Society of Gastrointestinal and Abdominal Radiology, Netherlands Association of Hepatogastroenterologists, Hellenic Society of Gastroenterology, Cardiovascular and Interventional Radiological Society of Europe, and Dutch Mesenteric Ischemia Study group clinical guidelines on the diagnosis and treatment of patients with chronic mesenteric ischaemia. United European Gastroenterol J. 2020;8(4):371–95. https://doi.org/10.1177/2050640620916681. Epub 2020 Apr 16. PMID: 32297566; PMCID: PMC7226699
4. Goodall R, Langridge B, Onida S, Ellis M, Lane T, Davies AH. Median arcuate ligament syndrome. J Vasc Surg. 2020;71(6):2170–6. https://doi.org/10.1016/j.jvs.2019.11.012.
5. Hanaki T, Fukuta S, Okamoto M, Tsuda A, Yagyu T, Urushibara S, Endo K, Suzuki K, Nakamura S, Ikeguchi M. Median arcuate ligament syndrome and aneurysm in the pancreaticoduodenal artery detected by retroperitoneal hemorrhage: a case report. Clin Case Rep. 2018;6(8):1496–500. https://doi.org/10.1002/ccr3.1643. PMID: 30147890; PMCID: PMC6099015
6. Chaer RA, Abularrage CJ, Coleman DM, Eslami MH, Kashyap VS, Rockman C, Murad MH. The Society for Vascular Surgery clinical practice guidelines on the management of visceral aneurysms. J Vasc Surg. 2020;72(1S):3S–39S. https://doi.org/10.1016/j.jvs.2020.01.039. Epub 2020 Mar 20
7. DeCarlo C, Woo K, van Petersen AS, Geelkerken RH, Chen AJ, Yeh SL, Kim GY, Henke PK, Tracci MC, Schneck MB, Grotemeyer D, Meyer B, DeMartino RR, Wilkins PB, Iranmanesh S, Rastogi V, Aulivola B, Korepta LM, Shutze WP, … Antonio S (2023) From the Society for Vascular Surgery Factors associated with successful median arcuate ligament release in an international, multi-institutional cohort. https://doi.org/10.1016/j.jvs.2022.10.022.
8. Jimenez JC, Harlander-Locke M, Dutson EP. Open and laparoscopic treatment of median arcuate ligament syndrome. J Vasc Surg. 2012;56(3):869–73. https://doi.org/10.1016/j.jvs.2012.04.057. Epub 2012 Jun 27
9. Reilly LM, Ammar AD, Stoney RJ, Ehrenfeld WK. Late results following operative repair for celiac artery compression syndrome. J Vasc Surg. 1985;2(1):79–91. https://doi.org/10.1016/0741-5214(85)90177-6.
10. Mouradian GP, Wessel E, Hance K, Hunter J. Isolated celiac artery avulsion from blunt abdominal trauma. Trauma Case Rep. 2023;46:100844. https://doi.org/10.1016/j.tcr.2023.100844. PMID: 37274543; PMCID: PMC10238870
11. Megalou A, Pantazopoulos IN, Antonopoulos CN, Argiriou M, Zakynthinos S, Mastora Z. Celiac artery avulsion secondary to blunt trauma: a case report. Ann Vasc Surg. 2017;43:314.e13–6. https://doi.org/10.1016/j.avsg.2017.02.018. Epub 2017 May 4

Chapter 15
Median Arcuate Ligament Syndrome in the Pediatric Population

Krysta M. Sutyak, Imad Absah, and Abdalla E. Zarroug

Introduction and Overview of Median Arcuate Ligament Syndrome

Median arcuate ligament syndrome (MALS) was first described by Lipshutz in 1917 [1]. Since its description, there has been controversy over the pathogenesis and the basis of its existence as a diagnosis for abdominal pain [2, 3]. The early publications and descriptions are of the adult population. It wasn't until the late twentieth century and early twenty-first century that we started to see descriptions in children and adolescents [4]. The questions around the existence of MALS as a true clinical syndrome are centered around the vague presentations and symptoms as well as the lack of consistent results, following surgical treatment in early studies [3, 5]. In the current literature, the diagnosis of MALS is supported, as is the surgical treatment of the disease with median arcuate ligament release, which has a reported improvement in symptoms between 70% and 80% in multiple retrospective reviews and case reports in pediatric patients [4].

Median arcuate ligament syndrome, also referred to as celiac artery compression syndrome, is known as a diagnosis of exclusion [2]. The presenting symptoms are colicky abdominal pain, nausea, and vomiting [1, 2]. These are relatively nonspecific and overlap with multiple other causes of abdominal pain, making the

K. M. Sutyak · A. E. Zarroug (✉)
Department of Surgery, University of Nebraska Medical Center, Omaha, NE, USA

Department of Surgery, Children's Nebraska, Omaha, NE, USA
e-mail: krysta.sutyak@unmc.edu; azarroug@childrensnebraska.org

I. Absah
Division of Pediatric Gastroenterology and Hepatology, Mayo Clinic, Rochester, MN, USA
e-mail: absah.imad@mayo.edu

D. Shouhed et al. (eds.), *Median Arcuate Ligament Syndrome*,
https://doi.org/10.1007/978-3-031-80740-4_15

diagnosis difficult to achieve [2]. There are some specific qualities to characterize the abdominal pain, which support the diagnosis of MALS, which includes postprandial and superior epigastric pain without radiation [1, 2, 6]. Reports include a wide variety of timing, including constant symptoms, symptoms 1–2 times a day, or a couple of times per month [6]. The duration of symptoms ranges from a couple of minutes to a number of hours. MALS in the pediatric population occurs the majority of the time in the female population, with most studies reporting upward of 80% of their patients as biologically female [1, 5–8]. While there are some outliers in the age reported in the literature as young as 3, the majority of patients were in their teenage years [6, 7, 9, 10]. Although anecdotal, the authors have found one unique feature associated with teenagers to be recurrent postexercise pain, much like the postprandial pain in adults; clinicians should ask about this in teenagers when considering MALS. Comorbid psychosocial diagnoses are common in children and adolescents undergoing workup for MALS as 50–75% of these patients have at least one diagnosis of an associated psychiatric condition [5, 8, 10]. However, we do not know if this is an independent factor or secondary, on some level, to having unexplained pain.

Chronic abdominal pain is a complex, frustrating, and common diagnosis in children [1]. Multiple diagnoses fall into this category, including functional gastrointestinal disorder, abdominal migraine, and IBS [1]. These particular patients have often undergone a multitude of tests and clinical exams with no proceeding diagnosis. Chronic abdominal pain can be very difficult for the patient, the family, and the treating provider as it leads to extensive workups, prohibitive healthcare costs, multiple visits to different medical providers, and the emergency room. The chronic abdominal pain disease burden comes with unique concerns to the pediatric patient population, such as absence from school and impacts on psychosocial and environmental development [2]. This is the population in which MALS should be suspected, and workup for MALS diagnosis should be considered.

The mainstay of treatment for the disease in the pediatric population is laparoscopic median arcuate ligament release. This is a safe and effective procedure that has been shown to increase the quality of life for children and adolescents with MALS and their families [1–4].

Special Considerations for the Pediatric Population

The discussion and evaluation of MALS in the pediatric population presents unique critical factors to assess when compared to the adult population. As with any diagnosis, and specifically those requiring surgical care when they occur in children, they alter different and additional lifestyle factors compared to adults. At the forefront of the care provided to the patient should be the child's experience and how it affects their development as a whole as well as the functioning of the family. The goal should be to optimize the child's experience given the presenting situation. It is worth perseverating on this point: the authors believe the goal of treatment is to improve the child's quality of life and not just relieve pain. Therefore, the ability to treat the compression with minimally invasive techniques plays a role in treatment decisions.

The associated psychological disorders present in about 50% of patients with a MALS diagnosis are of particular importance in children, as they occur during a period that is critical in overall development [5, 8]. For those who do not treat the pediatric population the majority of their time, it is crucial to understand that the growth and development of children are of paramount concern, something we don't need to consider in the adult population. Therefore, it is logical that anything that can delay or disrupt development should be considered, allowing the opportunity for the treatment team to discuss options with the patient and family.

The comorbid psychological disorders identified in the literature include mood disorders, such as depression, anxiety disorders, adjustment disorders, learning disorders, eating disorders, and rumination [1, 5, 8]. In addition to those diagnoses, children and adolescents with MALS have been identified to have poor coping mechanisms with a tendency for catastrophizing and helplessness [5, 8]. It is unclear at this time if the psychological symptoms developed secondary to the symptoms of MALS or were present before and despite the condition or what role the symptoms of MALS played in the potential worsening or exacerbation of underlying psychological symptoms [5, 8]. As such, a psychiatric or psychological evaluation is recommended as part of the multidisciplinary team approach during the workup and the decision of candidacy for surgery [1, 4, 5, 8].

If psychological diagnoses or symptoms are identified, it is recommended that the patient undergo treatment and optimization of this condition prior to any surgical treatment to optimize their postoperative experience [1, 5, 8]. However, previous studies assessing MALS and the psychosocial component suggest that the improved quality of life after surgical treatment and the absence or improvement of pain does not change the presence of the psychological symptoms or diagnoses [5, 8]. Lastly, it is important to consider the effect that a chronic abdominal pain diagnosis has on the child's life. In addition to the months to years of symptoms, they have undergone a multitude of doctor's visits, lab draws, imaging tests, and procedures [1, 5, 8, 10]. This leads to many missed school days from symptoms, limiting overall functioning and time for the above medical evaluation. In turn, this may allow the child to develop delays in learning and social issues with peers in the classroom. The sequela of these consequences has been shown to continue into adulthood [5]. The mainstay of preoperative management should focus on understanding and agreeing upon expectations for the hospital and postoperative course, optimization of underlying psychological diagnoses, and targeting maladaptive coping strategies. Current studies are investigating preoperative cognitive behavioral therapy to address these maladaptive mechanisms and teach healthy means of coping [5].

Diagnosis

Successful diagnosis and treatment of MALS include a multidisciplinary team, consisting of a pediatric gastroenterologist, a pediatric surgeon, a vascular surgeon, psychiatrist/psychologist, radiologist, pain specialists, and any other consulting service required for that particular patient [1–4, 6, 9–11]. The first step is a complete medical workup, which is often quite extensive [1, 3]. In the majority of cases, this has been completed prior to the patient's presentation to a MALS program or provider as they have a history of chronic abdominal pain over the prior months to years. The diagnostic algorithm is similar to that in adults (Fig. 15.1).

In the pediatric population, the recommended initial screening test for MALS is with a mesenteric duplex ultrasound [1–4, 6, 7, 9–11]. The main diagnostic measurement is the peak systolic velocity (PSV) of the celiac artery, with velocities greater than 200 cm/sec meeting criteria for compression [1, 3, 4] (Fig. 15.2).

The confirmatory test for MALS is with either CT or MR angiography (CTA or MRA), looking for the characteristic "J hook" (Figs. 15.3 and 15.4) appearance of the celiac artery, indicating compression [1–4, 6, 7, 9–11]. There is debate over which modality, CTA or MRA, is better in the pediatric population and currently varies by institution [1]. The major disadvantage of CT in the pediatric population is radiation exposure, especially in children who are medically complex and are at a higher likelihood of having had prior imaging or requiring future imaging [11]. It also involves the need for iodinated contrast material, and if a three-phased scan (rest, inhalation, exhalation) is performed, this may require more than one dose [11]. The advantage to CTA is that it is much quicker than MRA, which can be difficult in the pediatric population who are unable to perform the requirements for a high-quality MRI [10, 11]. In general, CT scans are also a more universally friendly imaging modality for all practitioners to review. The vascular anatomy and

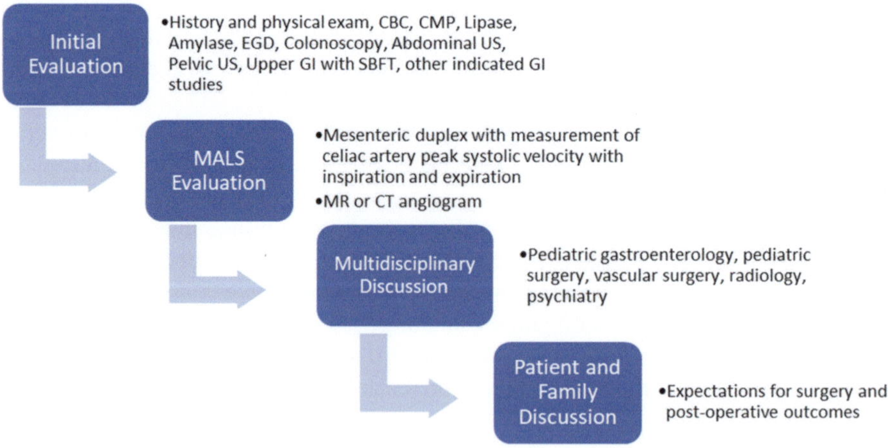

Fig. 15.1 Diagnostic algorithm

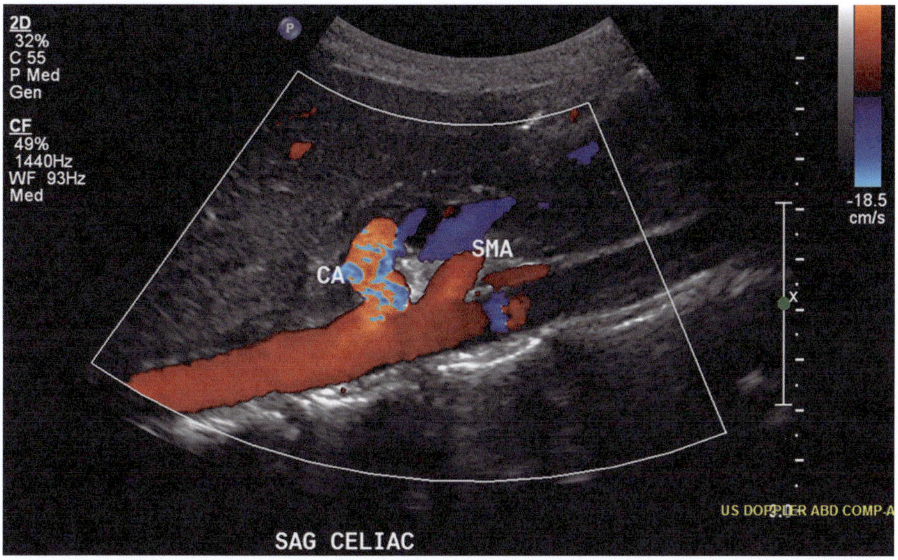

Fig. 15.2 Duplex US of the aorta, celiac artery (CA), and superior mesenteric artery (SMA)

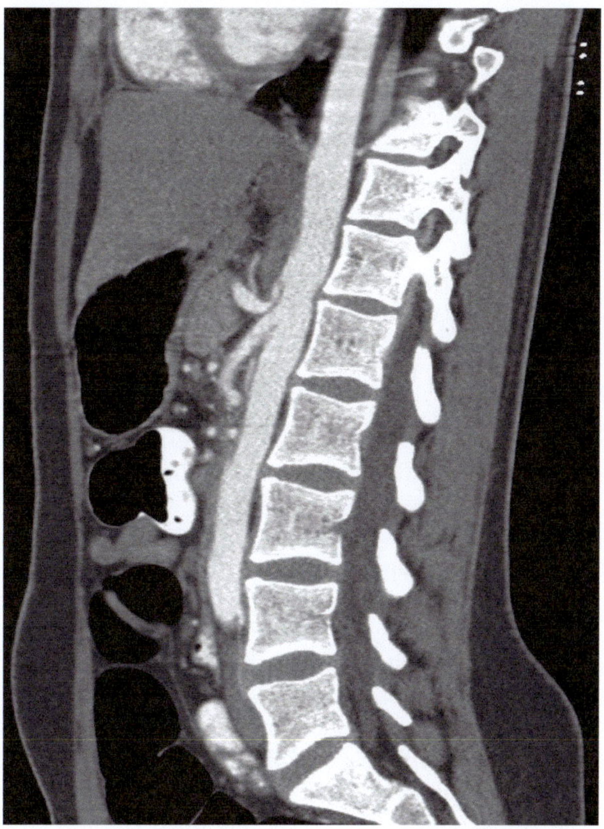

Fig. 15.3 MRA during expiration of a patient with MALS demonstrating the "J hook" configuration and narrowing at the celiac axis

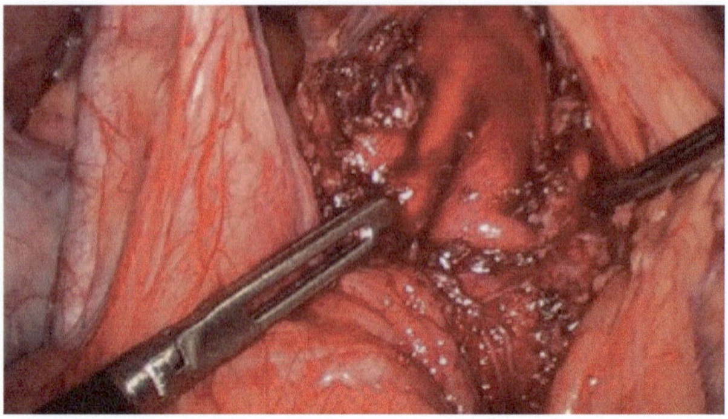

Fig. 15.4 Laparoscopic dissection visualizing the aorta and the celiac artery

surrounding relationships can be evaluated on MR, which is radiation-free, but there is a high risk for motion artifact if unable to remain still [10]. However, the majority of pediatric patients with MALS are in their teenage years and thus should be able to remain still for the required amount of time and follow any indicated directions [11]. Some argue the absence of radiation makes MR angiography preferred in the pediatric population [11].

Celiac plexus block has been suggested as an additional adjunct for diagnosis. When studied and implemented, patients received a block with 0.25% bupivacaine and were monitored [9]. They reported pain relief as soon as 30 min post-procedure with a duration of approximately 9 h [9]. A finding of pain relief supports the diagnosis of median arcuate ligament syndrome and may indicate success with surgical release and celiac ganglionectomy. However, this has not been widely implemented as part of the preoperative workup for diagnosis in children and adolescents, as it requires a procedure with sedation and the associated anesthesia and procedural risks [9, 10]. Celiac plexus blocks can be challenging and access to providers who perform this may be limited. We recommend referral to high-volume centers for evaluation and consideration.

Additionally, most centers that treat MALS patients feel the supporting evidence from the US and CT/MR angiography is sufficient. Celiac plexus block does play a role in the failure of pain relief postoperatively and may be a helpful adjunct where the imaging studies are non-diagnostic, but patients fit the symptom profile [10]. Furthermore, the authors have noticed anecdotally slightly more inflammatory tissue during the surgical release of MALS after some celiac plexus blocks.

Once the workup has been complete and the MALS specific imaging is supportive of the syndrome, a multidisciplinary decision should be made about the patient's candidacy for surgery [1, 3, 10, 12]. Any identified psychological symptoms should be optimized. Additionally, there may be a role for the pain team to discuss a pre- and postoperative pain plan [1]. The emphasis should be on reaching a consensus and understanding with the family. It is important to establish that this is an elective procedure with risks, and while it is successful in decreasing pain and increasing quality of life in 70–80% of patients, there are another 20–30% who do not have the desired outcome [1, 3, 8]. The informed consent process needs to occur using a shared decision-making process with the family and patient. We often have the family verbalize back to us what next steps the family will take after surgical release if the pain and symptoms do not go away.

Treatment

The operation for MALS is a median arcuate ligament release. This can be done open, laparoscopically, or robotically. The majority of MALS surgeons recommended concomitant neurolysis of the celiac plexus [1–4, 6, 10, 13]. The other point of discussion is the need for revascularization procedures at the time of intervention. In adults, endovascular approaches with angioplasty and stenting are being used for other forms of mesenteric ischemia, but they have not been found successful in MALS, likely secondary to external compression [1, 3].

The majority of pediatric MALS surgeons follow the technique outlined by Roayaie et al. with slight variations as needed to cater to the pediatric population [10]. The procedure is generally performed by a team consisting of a pediatric surgeon and a vascular surgeon [1–3, 10]. Cases are being done laparoscopically, robotically, or open.

Operative Technique

Here, we will describe the author's (AEZ) operative technique. The patient is positioned supine on the operating table in a split leg position or with stirrups to help facilitate a foregut dissection [3]. Five ports are used. A 5 mm or a 10 mm port is used at the umbilicus for the camera, depending on the size of the patient and the camera being used. A 10 mm 30-degree camera offers the best optics and angles to differentiate nerve fibers, muscle fibers, vascular structures, and other tissue. Four additional 5 mm ports are used, two on the left and two on the right (Fig. 15.5). The left lateral port is used for a liver retractor, which is crucial to visualization at the aortic hiatus, but a ventral retractor can also be used. The patient positioning and port alignment are similar to that done for pediatric Nissen fundoplication.

Once the abdomen is entered and insufflated, it should be meticulously explored for any other sources of abdominal pain [10]. Next, the gastrohepatic ligament is

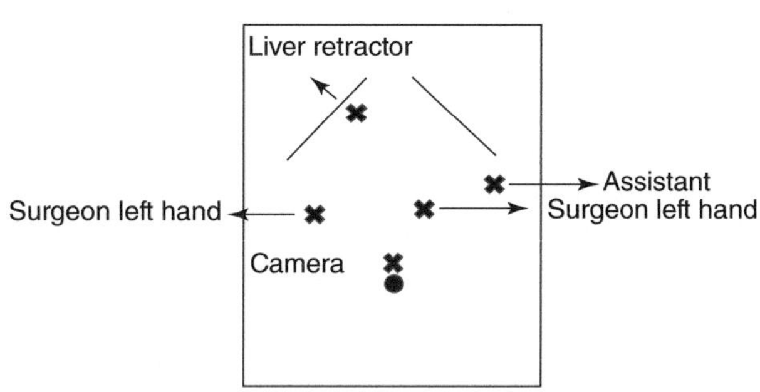

Fig. 15.5 Pediatric port placement diagram

opened and the right crus of the diaphragm is visualized [3]. The peritoneum over this structure is incised, allowing access to the retroesophageal space, which is bluntly and carefully developed [3]. The right and left crus of the aortic hiatus should be identified at this point. All of this so far should be bloodless. There are two ways to approach the crux of the dissection at the celiac axis. The first is to expose the aorta and then release the median arcuate ligament cranially to caudally along the anterior surface of the aorta [3]. The anterior surface is considered safe as there are no named branches until the celiac axis, and even with the numerous anatomical variants, staying truly anterior at 12 o'clock position is safe [3]. As the dissection moves cranially to caudally along the aorta, the celiac axis will be encountered and then can be skeletonized. The surgeon has to know the celiac axis will appear "hidden" at first as the median arcuate ligament is compressing it abnormally. Alternatively, the celiac axis can be approached in the opposite direction by starting dissection at the left gastric artery and following it to the celiac artery and eventually the aorta [3]. The author has attempted both approaches and has adopted the aortic to celiac dissection as their method of choice secondary to ease of the dissection in comparison to the gastric to celiac approach [3].

Along the dissection of the celiac axis, thin tight bands and nerve fibers will be encountered. These should be taken down one by one. The author prefers the L hook cautery, which allows for the identification of individual fibers and anterior traction of those fibers to lift them away from the aorta [3]. As the fibers are released, the celiac artery will begin to free, and outpouchings through the thick connective tissue will be visible. Dissection is continued in this fashion until the celiac axis is completely free circumferentially. The dissection is additionally carried out to 0.5–1.5 cm onto the common hepatic and the left gastric arteries [3]. This is the most important operative step, and it is imperative to the success of the operation that all fibers and bands are freed [1, 3]. Of note, the authors recommend against closing the crura with sutures [3]. This is supported by the experience of Mak et al. [10] who described an initial technique with full division of the crura and dissection from the esophageal hiatus to the aortic hiatus with re-approximation of the crura [10]. In their patient series, two individuals had postoperative esophageal symptoms requiring endoscopic intervention, so they adapted their technique and recommended minimal dissection at the hiatus [10]. Overall, the risk profile of this operation is low with the majority of complications being ongoing pain and nausea [1, 3, 10]. Lastly, blood and some kind of vascular patch should be available if technical complications occur.

Some authors describe the use of intraoperative ultrasound and measurement of the PSV in the celiac artery to confirm the release has been completed. However, others rely on the improved configuration of the celiac axis and the absence of all connective tissue material as the criteria for completion [1, 3]. If using intraoperative ultrasound, the criteria for complete release include normalization or significant reduction of the PSV of the celiac artery without changes in flow during the respiratory cycle [1, 10]. This is achieved by holding a Valsalva and measuring the PSV [1]. Revascularization procedures such as stenting or bypass are generally not performed at the index operation and are reserved as an option for treatment failure [1].

Based on the published success rates of median arcuate ligament release in symptom relief, around 20% of the patients will have continued pain postoperatively. It is recommended to have a plan for these patients ahead of time, given the reality that this situation may occur, and to have discussed this with the patient and family [1, 10]. If pain should persist or recur postoperatively, this should trigger a repeat evaluation with a mesenteric duplex and a CT or MR angiogram with repeat measurements of the celiac artery PSV and the other diagnostic information previously discussed [1, 10]. The patients will either have a normal PSV of the celiac artery with no change in flow during inspiration and expiration or continue to have abnormalities. For the patients who have elevated peak velocities of the celiac artery or respiratory variance despite surgical intervention, it is recommended they be considered for endovascular techniques such as stenting [10]. The reasoning for possible endovascular intervention postoperatively as opposed to preoperatively is that the external compression source has been relieved, so there should be no complications of stent compression or stenosis. In the patient population who have continued symptoms and normalization of the mesenteric duplex, celiac axis block should be considered [10].

Conclusion

Median arcuate ligament syndrome can be life-altering for children and adolescents. They have undergone extensive medical workup and have been living with chronic abdominal pain. Up to 20% of the pediatric population who have chronic abdominal pain characterize it as limiting daily functioning [5, 8]. While MALS is rare, from the literature, it does exist, and surgical treatment with laparoscopic median arcuate ligament release is effective in providing sustainable symptom relief in at least 70% of the patients [1, 4]. Additionally, psychological studies show that while comorbid conditions do not resolve, the patient-reported scores for physical functioning, mental health, self-esteem, general health perceptions, and quality of life are improved [3]. Workup for MALS should be considered in pediatric patients with chronic abdominal pain, consisting of a multidisciplinary approach, psychosocial support, and thorough shared decision-making with the patient and family surgical treatment may be offered.

References

1. Skelly C, Mak G. Median arcuate ligament syndrome—current state of management. Semin Pediatr Surg. 2021;30(6):151129.
2. Zarroug A. Diagnosis and treatment of MALS. Youtube, uploaded by Mayo Clinic, 3 May 2013. https://www.youtube.com/watch?v=EbFBaZRv558.
3. Joyce D, Antiel R, Oderich G, et al. Pediatric median arcuate ligament syndrome: surgical outcomes and quality of life. J Laparoendosc Adv Surg Tech. 2014;24(2):104–10.

4. Metz M, Blauw J, Brusse-Keizer M, et al. Systematic review of the efficacy of treatment for median arcuate ligament syndrome. Eur J Vasc Endovasc Surg. 2022;64:720–32.
5. Stiles-Shields C, Osos S, Heilbrun A, et al. Targeting coping to improve surgical outcomes in pediatric patients with median arcuate ligament syndrome: feasibility study. Front Psychol. 2021;12:695435.
6. Schweizer P, Berger S, Schweizer M, et al. Arcuate ligament vascular compression syndrome in infants and children. J Pediatr Surg. 2005;40:1616–22.
7. Klimas A, Lemmer A, Bergert H, et al. Laparoscopic treatment of celiac artery compression syndrome in children and adolescents. Vasa. 2015;44(4):305–12.
8. Stiles-Shields C, Skelly C, Mak G, et al. Psychological factors and outcomes in the surgical treatment of pediatric patients with median arcuate ligament syndrome. JPGN. 2018;66(6):866–71.
9. Selvaraj B, Joshi M, Weber G, et al. Celiac plexus block as a diagnostic tool in suspected pediatric median arcuate ligament syndrome. Local Reg Anesth. 2019;12:15–8.
10. Mak G, Speaker C, Anderson K, et al. Median arcuate ligament syndrome in the pediatric population. J Pediatr Surg. 2013;48(11):2261–70.
11. Aschenbach R, Basche S, Vogl T. Compression of the celiac trunk caused by median arcuate ligament in children and adolescent subjects: evaluation with contrast-enhanced MR angiography and comparison with Doppler US evaluation. J Vasc Interv Radiol. 2011;22:556–61.
12. Young-Chang A, Morimoto A, Sakurai H, et al. The effect of celiac plexus block on heart rate variability. J Anesth. 2013;1:62–5.
13. Gonzalez M, Balacco ME, Contreras S, et al. Videolaparoscopic management of arcuate ligament syndrome in pediatric patients. Cir Pediatr. 2021;34:47–50.

Chapter 16
Intraoperative and Early Postoperative Complications of Median Arcuate Ligament Release

Gustavo Romero-Velez, Juan S. Barajas-Gamboa, and Matthew Kroh

Introduction

Patient safety is one of the current priorities of the World Health Organization, which is of significant importance in the operating room, where surgeons need to remember the dictum *primum non nocere* [1, 2]. As healthcare systems shift to value-based models, it is necessary to optimize patient outcomes to achieve the best value in surgical care as complications are being carefully evaluated [3, 4]. Nonetheless, complications are inherent to surgical practice, and while some can be avoided, a substantial proportion of them are not preventable [5]. Surgeons need to pay particular attention to all potential complications for a given procedure during surgical planning.

Median arcuate ligament release (MALR) was first described in the 1960s by Harjola and Dunbar and remains the standard treatment for median arcuate ligament syndrome (MALS) [6, 7]. Although this is considered a rare condition, as Skelly et al. accurately pointed out, this is rather rarely diagnosed and treated [8]. As such, there is scarce but growing evidence with most of the data coming from case series. These are likely performed by surgeons with expertise in this complex disease and

G. Romero-Velez
Cleveland Clinic, Cleveland, OH, USA

J. S. Barajas-Gamboa
Cleveland Clinic Abu Dhabi, Abu Dhabi, UAE

M. Kroh (✉)
Cleveland Clinic Lerner College of Medicine of Case Western Reserve University, Digestive Disease Institute, Cleveland Clinic, Cleveland, OH, USA
e-mail: krohm@ccf.org

D. Shouhed et al. (eds.), *Median Arcuate Ligament Syndrome*,
https://doi.org/10.1007/978-3-031-80740-4_16

thus are prone to certain selection bias. In this chapter, we will describe the possible intraoperative as well as postoperative complications, which can guide surgeons in treating MALS during their surgical planning.

Intraoperative Complications

During any procedure, intraoperative complications can arise at different phases. These phases include the entry, retraction, dissection, resection, reconstruction, and closure [9]. As an abdominal procedure, MALR is prone to any of the complications inherent to laparotomy or laparoscopy, such as visceral/vascular injury during entry to the abdominal cavity or as a consequence of any other phase. A comprehensive review of all the possible intraoperative complications of laparotomy/laparoscopy is beyond the scope of this chapter and can be reviewed elsewhere. We will focus our attention on those complications specific to MALR.

Technical skills as well as anatomical knowledge are key components for a successful surgery [10]. As such, surgeons need to have a clear understanding of the structures at risk during any given operation. When approaching the target anatomy during MALR, because of the median arcuate ligament anatomic location, the most common structures at risk are the celiac trunk, including all its branches, the aorta, the inferior vena cava, the esophagus, the stomach, the pleura, and the liver [11]. Although intraoperative injuries are mostly identified during the operation, they can also present as an early complication in the postoperative period with a subsequent increase in morbidity, mortality, and length of stay [9, 12].

Of all structures at risk, intraoperative bleeding from vascular injury is of high importance and likely the most feared complication of MALR. Considering that the celiac trunk has a blood flow of 650 ml/min, injury to this vessel with uncontrolled bleeding would have a potentially fatal hemodynamic impact on patients in a matter of minutes [13]. Hence, as in any vascular procedure, it is fundamental to be able to achieve control, ideally both proximal and distal, during the operation. In addition and due to the high risk for vascular injury, traditionally MALR had been performed with an open approach, but since 2000, when the first laparoscopic approach was described, there has been increasing evidence of the safety of minimally invasive approaches, including both pure laparoscopic and robotic-assisted [14–16].

Minimally invasive MALR has proven to have equal long-term outcomes in terms of symptom improvement when compared to the standard of care, the open approach [17]. Although minimally invasive approaches for MALR appear to be increasing, certain factors need to be carefully reviewed when considering this type of approach [18]. First of all, the authors would suggest that this is only performed by advanced minimally invasive surgeons, preferably at centers with a comprehensive approach to MALS, including additional expertise in vascular surgery, gastrointestinal motility, pain management, and nutrition. In addition, surgeons performing minimally invasive MALR need to be conscious of the potential for conversion to open surgery. In our center experience, the conversion rate during the early learning curve was up to 10.3%, which dramatically decreased to no conversions during the last several years [15, 16]. This conversion rate is similar to that reported in a literature review, where a conversion rate of 9.1% was found mainly due to intraoperative bleeding [11]. For this reason, it is our institutional practice for MALR to be performed by a trained minimally invasive surgeon with immediate availability of a vascular surgeon if needed.

Interestingly, in one of the largest series of MALR, both the estimated blood loss (75 ml vs 50 ml, $p < 0.001$) and the rates of vascular injuries (3.5% vs 0.9%, $p = 0.06$) were lower during the laparoscopic approach. However, this higher estimated blood loss reported for the open approach is likely not clinically significant, in addition to the fact that patients who underwent an open approach had higher rates of concomitant mesenteric bypass (7.9% vs 0.0%, $p < 0.001$). On the other hand, in this study, the robotic approach was associated with the highest rates of vascular injury (5.6%), which the authors attributed to the early phases of the learning curve using the robotic platform [17]. In a similar way, a study using the American College of Surgeons-National Surgical Quality Improvement Project (ACS-NSQIP) database showed a significantly lower rate of intraoperative transfusions during the laparoscopic approach (7.5% vs 1.1%, $p < 0.001$) [18]. Regardless of the approach, surgeons doing MALR need to be aware of the potential risk of bleeding and plan for it, having type and cross available prior to the intervention.

In summary, major intraoperative bleeding during MALR appears to be a rare (2.5%) but potentially fatal complication. When attempting minimally invasive approaches, it is important to highlight that the small surgical field can rapidly fill with even small amounts of blood, making the exposure more challenging (Image 16.1). Having a gauze already in the surgical field to compress while adding extra ports can help achieve the minimally invasive approach. Other than careful dissection by experienced surgeons, we suggest having blood available prior to the intervention, an early threshold for conversion to an open approach when a minimally invasive approach is being attempted, and a collaborative approach between minimally invasive and vascular surgeons.

If a vascular injury occurs, as in any vascular procedure, proximal and distal control are needed to minimize bleeding while repairing the injury. Appropriate

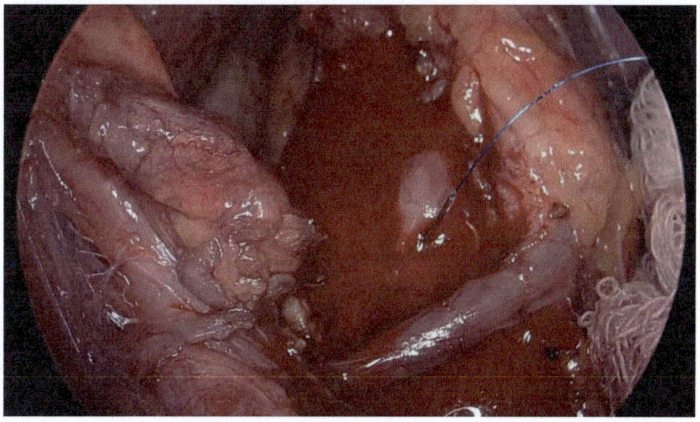

Image 16.1 Laparoscopic median arcuate ligament release complicated with intraoperative bleeding. The small surgical field fills rapidly with blood making the exposure challenging

intravenous access and arterial monitoring should be secured, based on patient characteristics. Additionally, open general and vascular surgery-specific instruments should be opened and immediately available if needed for urgent conversion, including appropriate sutures, for which we typically use 5-0 Prolene.

Visceral injuries are far less common than vascular injuries during MALR, reported in 0.2% of the cases with no differences between open and minimally invasive approaches [17]. As mentioned before, the liver, esophagus, and stomach are the most likely viscus injuries. The liver can be either directly injured with sharp or energy instruments during dissection, but it is also prone to capsular tear, parenchymal fracture, parenchymal congestion, and even parenchymal necrosis with the retractor and thus these should be kept in mind [19]. Finally, as the first step in exposing the celiac trunk is by dividing the pars flaccida of the hepatogastric ligament, surgeons approaching the celiac trunk need to be well aware of a ~ 10% prevalence of an accessory or replaced left hepatic artery in this area which, if ligated, can cause liver necrosis [20].

Another important complication related to MALR is capnothorax. Although frequently cited as a rare complication, capnothorax can be frequently found in upper abdominal procedures, especially in those with a close relationship to the diaphragm [21, 22]. As the right and left crus are dissected to expose the celiac trunk, there is always a possibility of damaging the pleura and creating a capnothorax. This manifests as hypoxemia, hypercapnia, and increased airway pressures. This complication is mostly self-limited as carbon dioxide is rapidly absorbed, and thus, it rarely requires tube thoracostomy to release the pressure. Nevertheless, this should be considered in cases in which hemodynamic instability is present [23].

Finally, when discussing potential intraoperative complications at the time of patient counseling, surgeons are usually confronted by patients asking for the risk of death during the operation. While patients presenting with MALS are mostly young and with a lower rate of concomitant comorbidities, there is always a risk during any type of surgery [17, 18]. MALR is considered a high intrinsic cardiac risk procedure, which confers a ~ 5% risk of nonfatal myocardial infarction or cardiac death based on perioperative risk stratification guidelines [24]. Even though it is difficult to account for the true incidence of death during MALR as those events are likely under reported in the literature, a recent study reported a 0.1% 30-day mortality risk in a 763 patient cohort during a 10-year period [18]. Therefore, it is likely that the overall risk might be lower than the 5% reported for high-risk procedures.

Early Complications

In a similar way to intraoperative complications, MALR is prone to any of the complications listed for abdominal surgery. These can range from wound complications to infectious complications or more serious cardiovascular complications. During surgical planning and patient counseling, surgeons frequently use the ACS-NSQIP risk calculator, which is a data-driven tool that can predict individual surgical risk based on clinical and operative variables [25]. However, as this tool utilizes a current procedural terminology (CPT) code to calculate the risk and there is no specific current CPT code for MALR, the tool might under or overestimate the surgical risk for a given patient [26].

In general, studies reporting operative outcomes for MALR cite low rates of 30-day complications but those mostly focus on major or MALR-specific complications [27–34]. Fortunately, two of the largest multicenter studies have confirmed such findings with a major complication rate of 3.1% [18]. In that study, the rate of major complications was significantly higher in the open approach, present in 4% of the cases compared to 0.5% in the laparoscopic approach. These major complications included organ space surgical site infection, reintubation, failure to wean, progressive renal insufficiency, stroke, cardiac arrest, myocardial infarction, septic shock, return to the operating room, and death. However, when looking at serious complications, such as myocardial infarction, cardiac arrest, and pulmonary embolism, there appears to be no difference between groups with fairly low occurrences [17, 18]. It has also been suggested by one study that open MALR is associated with higher rates of reoperation compared to the laparoscopic approach (2.6% vs 0%, $p = 0.03$), but others have failed to prove this difference between groups [17, 18].

In general, the rates of any 30-day complications have been cited to be between 10% and 20% [17, 18]. As mentioned before, these are not specific to MALR and include wound infections, postoperative pneumonia, deep vein thrombosis, and urinary tract infections, among others. In this regard, it is our practice to provide prophylactic antibiotics as well as perioperative subcutaneous heparin to patients as recommended by international guidelines to avoid these types of complications [35, 36]. A good proportion of this perioperative morbidity is due to a high incidence of ileus, which, as expected, is mostly associated with the open approach. The higher incidence of ileus also correlates with the fact that open MALR is reported to have longer lengths of stay in most published series [17, 18, 28, 37].

A rare but potential complication specific to MALR is injury to the cisterna chyli, which is usually located in the inter-aorto-caval space, just at the right of the aorta at the level of the celiac trunk. When encountered intraoperatively, this can be easily ligated or clipped (Image 16.2). If this structure is inadvertently injured

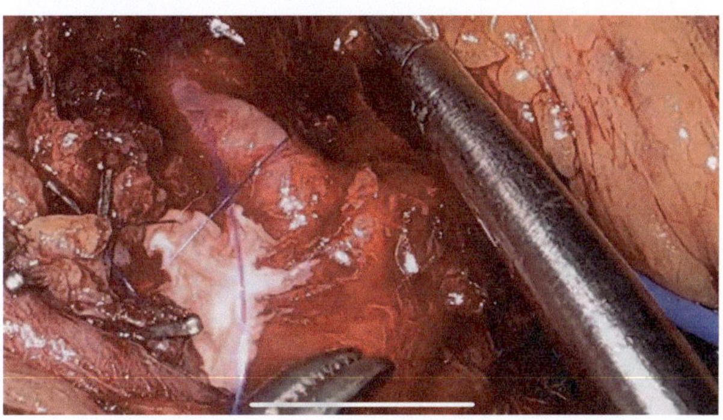

Image 16.2 Laparoscopic median arcuate ligament release complicated with chyle leak

during the operation, patients would present with nonspecific abdominal pain and will be found to have large volume ascites [38]. After paracentesis, the fluid has a typical milky appearance and should be tested for triglycerides, which if elevated confirms the diagnosis. First-line management is nonoperative with a high-protein low-fat diet to decrease the production of chyle [39]. In refractory cases of chylous ascites, percutaneous embolization of the lymphatic vessels has been described with good success rates [40]. Other options like external beam radiation have been described, but there is always the possibility that all of these measures fail and the surgeon is faced with the need to return and ligate the lymphatic leak [41].

Conclusions

Based on the available literature MALR appears to be an overall safe procedure. The open approach has been the standard of care since its description in the 1960s, the laparoscopic approach offers similar symptom improvement while having the advantage of lower rates of complications. Surgeons performing MALR should be familiar with the anatomy as there are specific complications related to the procedure such as major bleeding, capnothorax, and chylous ascites.

References

1. van Beuzekom M, Boer F, Akerboom S, Hudson P. Patient safety in the operating room: an intervention study on latent risk factors. BMC Surg. 2012;12(1):10. https://doi.org/10.1186/1471-2482-12-10.
2. Gifford RW. Primum non nocere. JAMA. 1977;238(7):589. https://doi.org/10.1001/jama.1977.03280070029018.
3. Porter ME, Teisberg EO. Redefining health care : creating value-based competition on results. Harvard Business School Press; 2006.
4. Leusder M, Porte P, Ahaus K, Van Elten H. Cost measurement in value-based healthcare: a systematic review. BMJ Open. 2022;12(12):e066568. https://doi.org/10.1136/bmjopen-2022-066568.
5. Healey MA, Shackford SR, Osler TM, Rogers FB, Burns E. Complications in surgical patients. Arch Surg. 2002;137(5):611–7.; discussion 617-618. https://doi.org/10.1001/archsurg.137.5.611.
6. Dunbar JD, Molnar W, Beman FF, Marable SA. Compression of the celiac trunk and abdominal angina: preliminary report of 15 cases. Am J Roentgenol. 1965;95(3):731–44. https://doi.org/10.2214/ajr.95.3.731.
7. Harjola PT, Lahtiharju A. Celiac axis syndrome. Am J Surg. 1968;115(6):864–9. https://doi.org/10.1016/0002-9610(68)90537-0.
8. Skelly CL, Mak GZ. Median arcuate ligament syndrome: surgical approaches to a rarely diagnosed and undertreated disease. J Vasc Surg. 2023;77(2):578–9. https://doi.org/10.1016/j.jvs.2022.11.046.
9. Mavros MN, Velmahos GC, Larentzakis A, et al. Opening Pandora's box: understanding the nature, patterns, and 30-day outcomes of intraoperative adverse events. Am J Surg. 2014;208(4):626–31. https://doi.org/10.1016/j.amjsurg.2014.02.014.

10. Clifton W, Damon A, Nottmeier E, Pichelmann M. The importance of teaching clinical anatomy in surgical skills education: spare the patient, use a sim! Clin Anat. 2020;33(1):124–7. https://doi.org/10.1002/ca.23485.
11. Jimenez JC, Harlander-Locke M, Dutson EP. Open and laparoscopic treatment of median arcuate ligament syndrome. J Vasc Surg. 2012;56(3):869–73. https://doi.org/10.1016/j.jvs.2012.04.057.
12. Bohnen JD, Mavros MN, Ramly EP, et al. Intraoperative adverse events in abdominal surgery: what happens in the operating room does not stay in the operating room. Ann Surg. 2017;265(6):1119–25. https://doi.org/10.1097/SLA.0000000000001906.
13. Kuntsevich GI, Shilenok DV. Duplex scanning of hemodynamic parameters of the celiac trunk and superior mesenteric artery in healthy volunteers. Khirurgiia (Mosk). 1993;7:48–51.
14. Roayaie S, Jossart G, Gitlitz D, Lamparello P, Hollier L, Gagner M. Laparoscopic release of celiac artery compression syndrome facilitated by laparoscopic ultrasound scanning to confirm restoration of flow. J Vasc Surg. 2000;32(4):814–7. https://doi.org/10.1067/mva.2000.107574.
15. Weber JM, Boules M, Fong K, et al. Median arcuate ligament syndrome is not a vascular disease. Ann Vasc Surg. 2016;30:22–7. https://doi.org/10.1016/j.avsg.2015.07.013.
16. Shin TH, Rosinski B, Strong A, et al. Robotic versus laparoscopic median arcuate ligament (MAL) release: a retrospective comparative study. Surg Endosc. Published online November. 2021;22 https://doi.org/10.1007/s00464-021-08877-1.
17. DeCarlo C, Woo K, van Petersen AS, et al. Factors associated with successful median arcuate ligament release in an international, multi-institutional cohort. J Vasc Surg. 2023;77(2):567–577.e2. https://doi.org/10.1016/j.jvs.2022.10.022.
18. Romero-Velez G, Barajas-Gamboa JS, Pantoja JP, et al. A nationwide analysis of median arcuate ligament release between 2010 and 2020: a NSQIP study. Surg Endosc. 2023;37(1):140–7. https://doi.org/10.1007/s00464-022-09431-3.
19. Tamhankar AP, Kelty CJ, Jacob G. Retraction-related liver lobe necrosis after laparoscopic gastric surgery. JSLS. 2011;15(1):117–21. https://doi.org/10.4293/108680811X13022985131651.
20. Yamamoto M, Zaima M, Yamamoto H, et al. Liver necrosis shortly after pancreaticoduodenectomy with resection of the replaced left hepatic artery. World J Surg Oncol. 2017;15(1):77. https://doi.org/10.1186/s12957-017-1151-2.
21. Wu Q, Zhang H. Carbon dioxide pneumothorax following retroperitoneal laparoscopic partial nephrectomy: a case report and literature review. BMC Anesthesiol. 2018;18(1):202. https://doi.org/10.1186/s12871-018-0662-x.
22. Msezane LP, Zorn KC, Gofrit ON, Schade GR, Shalhav AL. Case report: conservative management of a large capnothorax following laparoscopic renal surgery. J Endourol. 2007;21(12):1445–7. https://doi.org/10.1089/end.2007.0122.
23. Phillips S, Falk GL. Surgical tension pneumothorax during laparoscopic repair of massive hiatus hernia: a different situation requiring different management. Anaesth Intensive Care. 2011;39(6):1120–3. https://doi.org/10.1177/0310057X1103900621.
24. Fleisher LA, Fleischmann KE, Auerbach AD, et al. 2014 ACC/AHA guideline on perioperative cardiovascular evaluation and management of patients undergoing noncardiac surgery: a report of the American College of Cardiology/American Heart Association Task Force on practice guidelines. J Am Coll Cardiol. 2014;64(22):e77–137. https://doi.org/10.1016/j.jacc.2014.07.944.
25. Cohen ME, Ko CY, Bilimoria KY, et al. Optimizing ACS NSQIP modeling for evaluation of surgical quality and risk: patient risk adjustment, procedure mix adjustment, shrinkage adjustment, and surgical focus. J Am Coll Surg. 2013;217(2):336–46e1. https://doi.org/10.1016/j.jamcollsurg.2013.02.027.
26. Roddy SP. Laparoscopic versus open celiac ganglionectomy in patients with median arcuate ligament syndrome. J Vasc Surg. 2010;52(5):1419. https://doi.org/10.1016/j.jvs.2010.09.030.
27. El-Hayek KM, Titus J, Bui A, Mastracci T, Kroh M. Laparoscopic median arcuate ligament release: are we improving symptoms? J Am Coll Surg. 2013;216(2):272–9. https://doi.org/10.1016/j.jamcollsurg.2012.10.004.

28. Diab J, Diab V, Berney CR. A diagnostic workup and laparoscopic approach for median arcuate ligament syndrome. ANZ J Surg. Published online February 2022:ans.17514. doi:https://doi.org/10.1111/ans.17514.
29. Pather K, Kärkkäinen JM, Tenorio ER, et al. Long-term symptom improvement and health-related quality of life after operative management of median arcuate ligament syndrome. J Vasc Surg. 2021;73(6):2050–8.e4. https://doi.org/10.1016/j.jvs.2020.10.074.
30. van Petersen AS, Vriens BH, Huisman AB, Kolkman JJ, Geelkerken RH. Retroperitoneal endoscopic release in the management of celiac artery compression syndrome. J Vasc Surg. 2009;50(1):140–7. https://doi.org/10.1016/j.jvs.2008.12.077.
31. Roberts B, Pevsner R, Alkhoury F. Robotic approach for median arcuate ligament release in pediatrics. J Laparoendosc Adv Surg Tech. 2020;30(1):92–6. https://doi.org/10.1089/lap.2019.0337.
32. Fernstrum C, Pryor M, Wright GP, Wolf AM. Robotic surgery for median arcuate ligament syndrome. JSLS. 2020;24(2):e2020.00014. https://doi.org/10.4293/JSLS.2020.00014.
33. Coelho JCU, Hosni AVE, Claus CM, et al. Treatment of median arcuate ligament syndrome: outcome of laparoscopic approach. ABCD, arq bras cir dig. 2020;33(1):e1495. https://doi.org/10.1590/0102-672020190001e1495.
34. Sultan SA, Acharya Y, Mustafa M, Hynes N. Two decades of experience with chronic mesenteric ischaemia and median arcuate ligament syndrome in a tertiary referral centre: a parallel longitudinal comparative study. Cureus. Published online December. 2021;27 https://doi.org/10.7759/cureus.20726.
35. Anderson DR, Morgano GP, Bennett C, et al. American Society of Hematology 2019 guidelines for management of venous thromboembolism: prevention of venous thromboembolism in surgical hospitalized patients. Blood Adv. 2019;3(23):3898–944. https://doi.org/10.1182/bloodadvances.2019000975.
36. Bratzler DW, Dellinger EP, Olsen KM, Perl TM, Auwaerter PG, Bolon MK, Fish DN, Napolitano LM, Sawyer RG, Slain D, Steinberg JP, Weinstein RA.Clinical practice guidelines for antimicrobial prophylaxis in surgery. American Society of Health-System Pharmacists (ASHP); Infectious Diseases Society of America (IDSA); Surgical Infection Society (SIS); Society for Healthcare Epidemiology of America (SHEA).Surg Infect (Larchmt). 2013;14(1):73–156. https://doi.org/10.1089/sur.2013.9999. Epub 2013 Mar 5.
37. Birkhold M, Khalifeh A, Nagarsheth K, Kavic SM. Median arcuate ligament syndrome is effectively relieved with minimally invasive surgery. JSLS. 2022;26(4):e2022.00067. https://doi.org/10.4293/JSLS.2022.00067.
38. Sakai L, Aguilera P, Karmegam S. Acute chylous ascites status post median arcuate ligament syndrome decompression: a unique case report and literature review. Cureus. 2023;15(2):e35300. https://doi.org/10.7759/cureus.35300.
39. Santos E, Moussa AM. Chylous ascites and lymphoceles: evaluation and interventions. Semin Intervent Radiol. 2020;37(3):274–84. https://doi.org/10.1055/s-0040-1713445.
40. Cope C, Kaiser LR. Management of unremitting chylothorax by percutaneous embolization and blockage of retroperitoneal lymphatic vessels in 42 patients. J Vasc Interv Radiol. 2002;13(11):1139–48. https://doi.org/10.1016/s1051-0443(07)61956-3.
41. Kim SW, Kim JH. Low-dose radiation therapy for massive chylous leakage after subtotal gastrectomy. Radiat Oncol J. 2017;35(4):380–4. https://doi.org/10.3857/roj.2017.00178.

Chapter 17
Long-Term Outcomes After Surgery Including Recurrent Median Arcuate Ligament Syndrome

Jamie DeCicco and Kevin El-Hayek

Introduction

Surgery is the most common intervention used to treat median arcuate ligament syndrome (MALS). Response to surgery can vary widely among patients. In those with a positive response, some patients respond quickly and have immediate relief, while others have a longer recovery and gradually improve over time. Most studies report symptom improvement in roughly 80% of patients after MALS surgery, with studies ranging from 70% to 90% improvement during follow-up periods of 30 days to 6 months [1–5]. Of the 10–30% of patients who do not improve, individuals may have residual MALS with unresolved symptoms, recurrent MALS in which they had initial relief, but symptoms returned, or another reason for their presentation. The delineation of expectations cannot be emphasized enough as not all gastrointestinal symptoms are expected to resolve after surgery for MALS. The chief complaint that should be discussed and targeted is postprandial or post-exertional epigastric pain. Estimations for each of these categories have not been established.

J. DeCicco (✉)
Cleveland Clinic Lerner College of Medicine of Case Western Reserve University, Cleveland, OH, USA

Division of General Surgery, Department of Surgery, The MetroHealth System, Cleveland, OH, USA

K. El-Hayek
Department of Surgery, The MetroHealth System, Case Western Reserve University School of Medicine, Cleveland, OH, USA
e-mail: Kelhayek@metrohealth.org

D. Shouhed et al. (eds.), *Median Arcuate Ligament Syndrome*,
https://doi.org/10.1007/978-3-031-80740-4_17

Long-Term Outcomes

While research on MALS is generally limited, data on long-term outcomes after surgical intervention is even more scarce. There are some studies that report outcomes a few years after surgery, which provide more insight into the lasting effects of the intervention. Pather et al. investigated outcomes in adult patients who had undergone open or laparoscopic MAL release with a mean follow-up of 8 ± 4 years [6]. Initially, 83% of patients reported symptom improvement shortly after surgery, consistent with average outcomes in shorter-term studies [6]. At 12 months, however, 63% of patients reported symptom improvement or resolution and 37% reported unchanged symptoms [6]. After 5 years, this pattern seemed to persist in those patients who followed up, with 65% having symptom improvement compared to before surgery and 35% having continued symptoms [6]. This may indicate that status at the 1-year mark is a good indicator of prognosis after surgery, although more studies are needed to support this claim [6]. Additionally, this study was done only on patients who underwent MAL release, and other studies have shown that celiac ganglion resection may assist in achieving relief for a higher percentage of patients [7]. A systemic review that included studies with celiac artery release, celiac plexus resection, or celiac plexus blockage helped to characterize outcomes after any MALS intervention [5]. The review consisted of 38 studies describing 880 adult patients and six studies describing 195 pediatric patients [5]. It found symptom relief for more than 70% of patients from 3 to 228 months postop for adults and 6 to 62 months postop for pediatrics [5]. While this does not delineate between the interventions and has a wide range of follow-up, it may indicate that celiac ganglionectomy helps increase the percentage of patients with symptom improvement.

Variables Influencing Outcomes

The prognosis for patients with MALS varies depending on a variety of factors, including but not limited to type, severity, and duration of symptoms, comorbidities, and effectiveness of interventions used. Some studies have attempted to identify these factors that predict outcomes of surgical treatment. Ho et al. compared 67 patients, 43 with surgical intervention (open or laparoscopic MAL release) and 24 with conservative management, and a median follow-up of 2 years [8]. They found patients with exercise-induced or post-exertional pain were more likely to improve with surgery, whereas patients with vomiting and unprovoked pain had less favorable outcomes [8]. Birkhold et al. also found that other medical conditions, including psychiatric disorders and patients requiring additional vascular interventions, had less favorable outcomes [9]. Alternatively, a study by Reilly et al. with a mean follow-up of 9 years reported good surgical outcomes were correlated with female sex, younger age, postprandial abdominal pain, significant weight loss (>9 kg), lack of psychiatric history, and catheter angiographic features of post-stenotic dilation and increased collateral flow [10]. These factors may be associated with better outcomes because they are more specific to MALS, compared to other comorbidities that may present similarly or have symptom overlap, and suggest the surgery is specifically addressing the cause of their symptoms.

In cases where there is a long time to diagnose and high severity of symptoms, the chronic compression of the celiac artery may result in reduced blood flow to the gastrointestinal (GI) tract, possibly leading to tissue damage and additional complications. Additionally, chronic compression of the celiac ganglia may influence symptom resolution. Like other conditions involving nerve compression, hypersensitivity may develop, making it more difficult to break the cycle of pain even after proper surgical decompression has occurred. However, there is typically sufficient collateral blood flow, and other factors are likely contributing to the complex symptom presentation in these patients. A potential complication of prolonged compromised blood flow may be tissue damage and dysfunction, as several patients have issues with other parts of their GI tract. This is just one hypothesis, however, because there is typically sufficient collateral blood flow, and other factors could be contributing to this pan-dysmotility. Recent research on glial cells in the GI tract has revealed roles in digestion, nutrient absorption, blood flow, and immune responses [11, 12]. Dysfunction of these cells can create inflammatory responses, hypersensitization of neurons, and alter motility [13, 14]. Further study of the role of glial cells in patients with MALS may be a promising area of future investigation. Other factors contributing to symptoms may include tissue structure, such as defective collagen production as in Ehlers-Danlos syndrome (EDS), or issues with nervous tissue signaling. Compromised blood flow to the GI tract may also affect its ability to properly absorb nutrients, further contributing to malnutrition and weight loss. Significant weight loss due to MALS and loss of the mesenteric fat pad around the superior mesenteric artery can lead to other compression syndromes, including superior mesenteric artery syndrome (SMAS) and nutcracker syndrome (NCS).

Because patients often have multiple comorbidities, it is important to work with a multidisciplinary team to address other factors that may influence their response to surgery and overall health. Pediatric and young adult female patients seem to be especially at risk for numerous health conditions, including psychiatric concerns [15, 16], compression syndromes as discussed in Chap. 8, and the trifecta of postural orthostatic tachycardia syndrome (POTS), mast cell activation syndrome (MCAS), and EDS as discussed in Chap. 7. Beyond treatment for these conditions, additional interventions to manage symptoms such as pain management, dietary modifications, and mental health services are imperative in supporting any surgical operation to optimize the patient's strength, recovery, and mental health. See Chap. 9 for a more detailed discussion on nonoperative management.

Finally, the approach to surgery may impact a patient's recovery and overall surgical response. The advantages and disadvantages of each approach, including open, laparoscopic, and robotic, are discussed in more detail in Chaps. 10, 11, and 12. These chapters comment on morbidity and recovery of the procedure and how the artery and nerves are or are not addressed during the operations, expanding on the comments made in this chapter.

If a patient does not respond optimally to primary surgery, residual or recurrent MALS or an alternative diagnosis may be of interest to investigate. In such cases, clear and realistic expectations need to be communicated to the patient based on their anatomy, comorbidities, treatment options, risks, benefits, and outcomes of reoperation. Surgeons and physicians involved in the patient's care should make recommendations in the best interest of that specific patient, ultimately with the patient as the primary driver of their health decisions.

Role of Testing

Preoperative and postoperative imaging may help predict a patient's response to surgery. Some surgeons recommend repeating the mesenteric duplex ultrasound, typically 1–3 months postoperatively, to evaluate changes in velocities as a result of the primary operation. If symptoms persist or recur after this time frame, ultrasound velocities may also be obtained. A model based on 42 patients post-laparoscopic MAL release with a mean follow-up of 28.5 ± 18.8 months supports that age and baseline celiac artery expiratory velocity are significant predictors of quality-of-life improvement [17]. The model suggests that lower baseline velocities are associated with better outcomes, which may be because lower velocities typically indicate less severe compression. However, there is opposing evidence from other studies in which patients with more severe occlusion of the celiac trunk (>70%) had better results from surgery, with complete resolution of symptoms in 71% of cases [18]. This may be because the operation is relieving the compression contributing to symptoms. Similarly, DeCicco et al. found that a greater decrease in pre- to postoperative celiac artery velocities was associated with a positive response to surgery [7]. Therefore, it is important to note that ultrasound velocities are simply a marker for compression improvement or relief. If a patient still has high postoperative ultrasound velocities (≥200 cm/s), it does not necessarily mean the operation was unsuccessful. Any decrease in velocity is usually a sign of improvement, and some patients may simply have higher velocities at baseline. Additionally, if a patient's symptoms improve but velocities are persistently high, the treating physician may need to reassure the patient of their progress, mindful to treat the patient, not the test. There may be some cases, however, where a patient's symptoms continue or return after surgery, and there is corresponding diagnostic evidence on mesenteric duplex ultrasound. Such patients may fall into two categories: patients who never had symptom relief either from an alternative diagnosis or not a full release, consistent with residual MALS, or patients who had symptom relief for a period of time, but have return of symptoms +/− scarring, consistent with recurrent MALS. Other tests that may be done to evaluate for persistent or recurrent compression include repeat angiography (computerized tomography angiography (CTA) or magnetic resonance angiography (MRA)) to visualize the vasculature and repeat celiac plexus block with relief of symptoms. When evaluating a patient for residual or recurrent MALS after a primary operation, the surgeon should review the operative report from the initial operation. In some practices, a completed MAL release (+/− celiac ganglionectomy and lymphadenectomy) operative photo is placed in the chart or given to the patient, which should also be reviewed by the surgeon. In cases where the evaluating surgeon differs from the surgeon who performed the primary operation, reaching out to discuss their case and details of the operation may be helpful.

Many of the variables that influence outcomes of primary surgery may contribute to residual and recurrent MALS.

Residual MALS

There are several potential reasons for lack of response to surgery or residual symptoms after surgery. To be a surgical candidate, patients should have evidence of celiac artery and ganglia compression preoperatively based on ultrasound and/or CTA or MRA findings. If a MAL release was done during the operation but postoperative ultrasound or imaging never showed relief of the compression, there may have been an inadequate or incomplete release of the median arcuate ligament. This may be due to the surgeon's experience and competency in performing the operation. Some patients' anatomy may also be difficult to navigate and pose challenges in completing the release. For example, patient X was evaluated for candidacy to undergo a second operation after the first one was unsuccessful in relieving symptoms. A careful preoperative review of all imaging was done, and the patient's case was discussed with a multidisciplinary team to plan for the steps during the operation, prevent emergent conversion, and optimize surgical success (Fig. 17.1). Upon

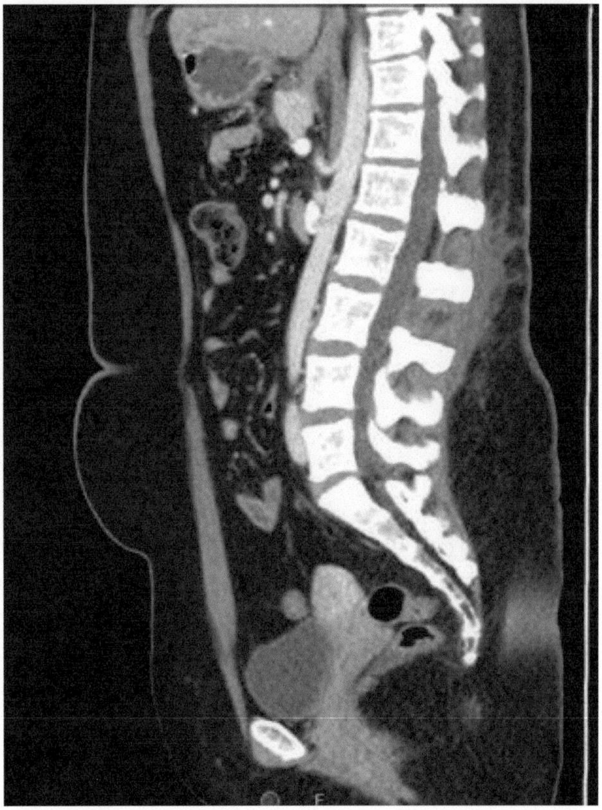

Fig. 17.1 Sagittal view of patient X anatomy on CTA used for preoperative planning. Low celiac takeoff and infrapancreatic view (below the splenic vein) are visualized

intraoperative exploration, the patient had severe adhesions from previous hiatal dissection requiring greater than 2 hours of lysis of adhesions to access the hiatus. The celiac trunk was compressed by the median arcuate ligament, confirmed by intraoperative ultrasound (Fig. 17.2). Furthermore, the patient's celiac trunk emanated from an infrapancreatic portion of the aorta, making it difficult to access (Fig. 17.3). An infrapancreatic dissection was required with additional release from the inferior aspect of the celiac artery and division of the left gastric vein superiorly (Fig. 17.4) until complete release with celiac ganglionectomy and lymphadenectomy was achieved (Fig. 17.5). A video review was also conducted after the operation to assess what went well and what could be improved for similar cases in the future. The surgeon who performed this redo operation has expertise in operating on pancreatic pathologies in addition to a high number of MALS and MALS redo cases; as such, they felt well-equipped to address this patient's case. Surgeons or centers with less experience may not feel comfortable treating this type of patient and have concerns about conversion or causing more harm. If this is the case,

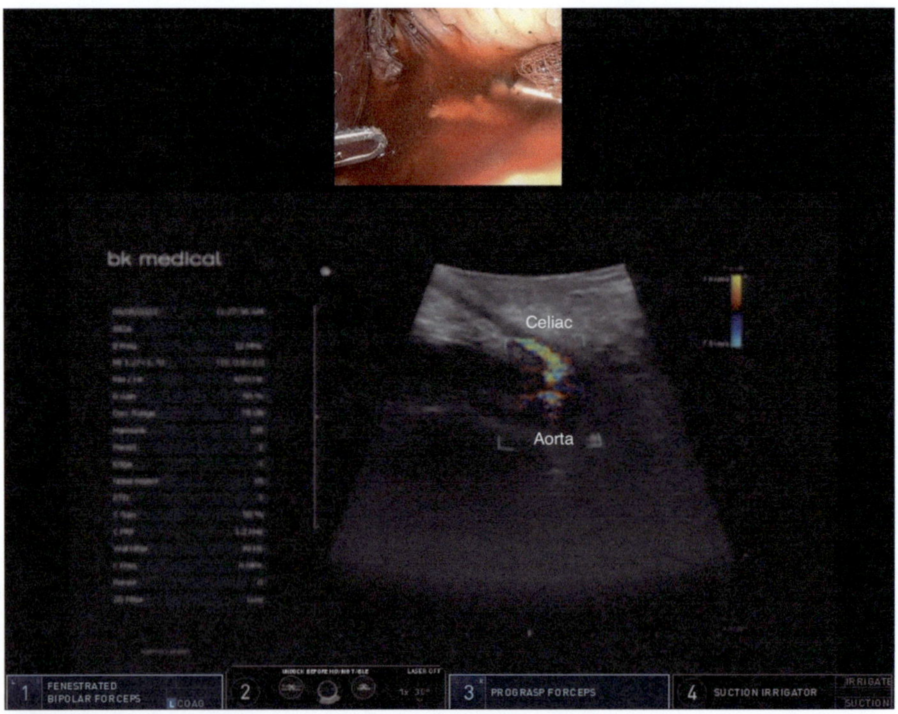

Fig. 17.2 Prerelease ultrasound of patient X demonstrating compression of the celiac artery via the MAL

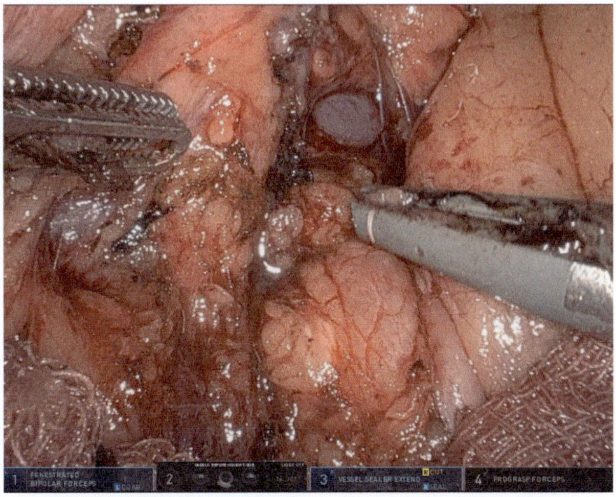

Fig. 17.3 Infrapancreatic approach to MAL release for patient X. Pancreas is superior to the splenic vein

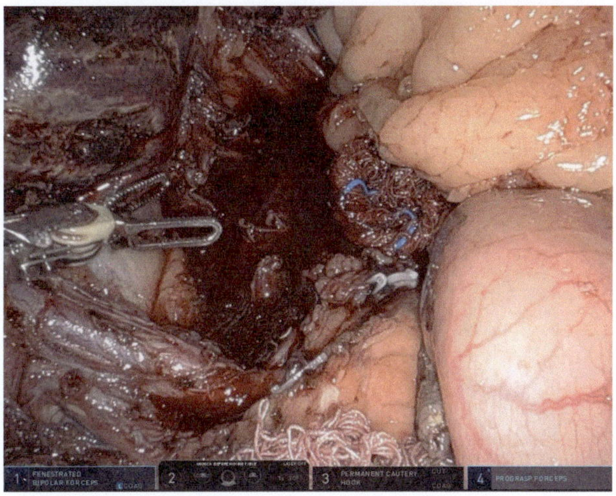

Fig. 17.4 Left gastric vein division in patient X

collaborations and/or referrals may be in the best interest of the patient and surgeon. With the level of patient complexity, variations in anatomy, and a high-risk operating region near the abdominal aorta, MALS cases should be carefully reviewed beforehand and multidisciplinary or even multicenter collaboration considered to provide the best chance at a successful outcome for these patients.

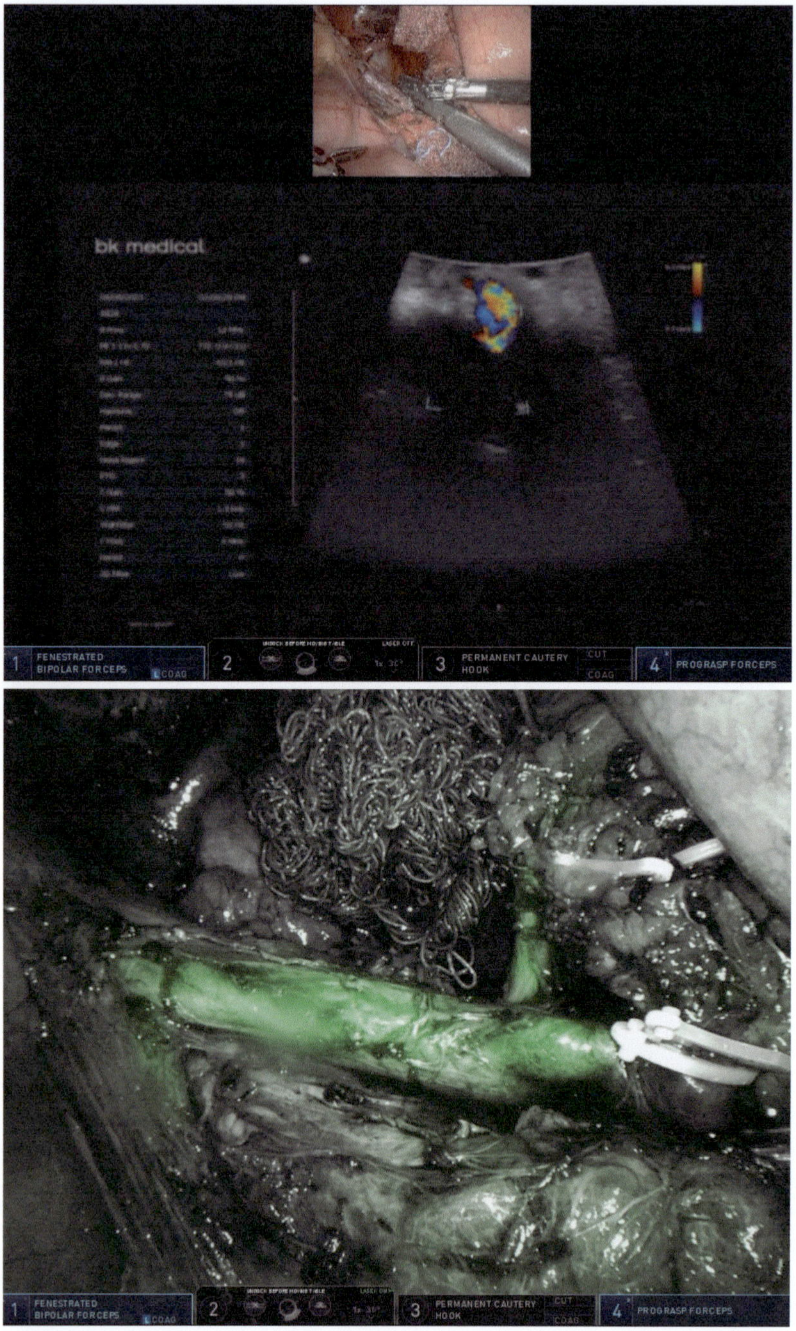

Fig. 17.5 Post-release ultrasound demonstrating improved blood flow through the celiac artery and visualization of vasculature via ICG for patient X

Recurrent MALS

Another category of patients may have recurrent MALS with temporary relief of symptoms after the initial operation, but symptoms return. There are reports of these cases in the literature, but data is limited based on patient follow-up.

Operative Concerns

One reason for symptom recurrence may be due to inadequate alleviation of arterial compression, and some surgeons employ follow-up vascular interventions to augment release. In a study of 13 patients undergoing laparoscopic MAL release with a median follow-up of 117 (45–185) months, Cienfuegos et al. found that nine patients had early full symptom resolution after surgery [18]. However, two of these patients experienced a recurrence of symptoms at 24 and 70 months post-op, undergoing subsequent angioplasty and stent placement [18]. Four patients did not have relief from surgery at all with persistent symptoms, falling into the residual category [18]. In another study of 21 patients undergoing laparoscopic MAL release, 18 (81%) patients had immediate postoperative symptom improvement [19]. However, seven (33%) of these patients had recurrent symptoms with persistent celiac stenosis and underwent subsequent percutaneous transluminal angioplasty with celiac stent placement around 50 days postoperatively [19]. Two of these patients failed endovascular intervention and required surgical bypass [19]. Overall, angioplasty and stent placement may be a helpful adjunct to surgery in some cases, but these interventions have limitations as they do not address the underlying extrinsic compression that results in symptoms [20].

Another reason for residual or recurrent MALS could be if a MAL release only was performed during the operation. With increasing evidence for the celiac ganglion playing a role in MALS symptoms, patients may need an anterior celiac ganglion resection to achieve symptom improvement [7]. In a study comparing laparoscopic and robotic MALS in 16 patients, three patients had recurrence of symptoms after laparoscopic surgery and one after robotic [21]. Two were treated with percutaneous transluminal angioplasty and stent placement and had continual symptoms after surgery, despite no recurrent celiac artery stenosis on postoperative imaging, suggesting there may be another reason for their symptoms [21]. One of these patients did have relief with subsequent celiac plexus blocks, suggesting the celiac ganglion was not appropriately addressed during surgery and may have been necessary to achieve symptom resolution. In another study by Weber et al., six out of 26 patients who underwent follow-up duplex ultrasound imaging after MAL release and plexus cauterization showed persistent stenosis and one occlusion but were symptom-free [22]. This finding suggests an important role of the nerve plexus fibers and the possibility that release and cauterization of the plexus fibers may be sufficient in some cases to relieve symptoms. Therefore, patients with residual or recurrent MALS may benefit from revision surgery. The goal is aimed at addressing persistent or recurrent symptoms after a previous MALS operation to improve symptoms, correct previously unaddressed issues, and improve quality of life. Recurrent MALS symptoms after surgical release have been shown in some studies to be safely treated with laparoscopic re-exploration [23]. Strong et al. found that the presence of persistent fibrous tissue and celiac plexus appeared to explain recurrent symptoms, and complete neurolysis may allow for favorable results with symptomatic relief [24]. However, there are very few reports of revision cases. Our group has preliminary data on ten patients, all with safe outcomes, but only 50% had relief of symptoms after reoperation. Those who did not have improvement often had multiple medical comorbidities (multiple compressions, POTS, MCAS, EDS/HSD) and a history of smoking and/or opioid medication use. Overall, more data is needed to comment on the risks, benefits, and outcomes of reoperation.

Medical Concerns

One reason for recurrence may be a buildup of scar tissue in the area surgical release was performed where the median arcuate ligament was compressing the celiac artery. MALS has also been associated with Ehlers-Danlos syndrome (EDS), predisposing patients to difficult wound healing and may be more likely to have post-surgical complications and abnormal scarring [25]. Most of these patients have hypermobile EDS, and there is still much unknown about this condition, its cause, and its impact on tissues. Often, atrophic scarring is seen in EDS, as there is more disorganized tissue and weaker tissue integrity [26]. This can result in poor healing, and the tissue that does form may be more distensible, fibrotic, and less structurally sound, leading to laxity and damage to surrounding structures. There have been reports of hypertrophic scarring as well, with extra aberrant connective tissue forming at the site of tissue injury [27]. This buildup of scar tissue may result in subsequent recompression of the celiac artery. Therefore, the approach to surgery should be taken into consideration when choosing how to operate. Patients with EDS may do better with a minimally invasive laparoscopic or robotic approach as opposed to an open approach, given that there is less risk for scar tissue formation.

Continued or recurrent symptoms may also occur because MALS overlaps with several other complex conditions that may contribute to symptoms and/or mimic MALS pain. In addition to EDS, other compression syndromes, including SMAS, NCS, and May-Thurner syndrome (MTS) as discussed in Chap. 8, and other medical conditions, including POTS, MCAS, gastroparesis, and other GI motility disorders as discussed in Chap. 7, may be contributing. For example, a patient who failed to get relief after MAL release and stent placement was eventually diagnosed with gastroparesis and had a gastric electrical stimulator placed for the resolution of symptoms [23]. Psychiatric conditions may also play a role in how a patient responds to surgery and their clinical outcomes [16]. Interventions addressing mental health conditions and the medical trauma these patients have been through while teaching effective coping strategies have been effective in improving pain and outcomes postoperatively [23].

A common theme in multiple studies is that most patients would still choose to undergo their primary operation if given the option to go back in time, even if they had symptom recurrence [6, 28]. This may be because patients had symptom relief for a brief period, or symptom severity improved after surgery; however, this is yet to be characterized. Additional investigation and questionnaires are needed to understand the reason for their answers.

Final Management Recommendations

Considering the data presented in this chapter, patients should be well informed about the outcomes of MALS surgery, as well as rates specific to their treating surgeon and the surgical approach used, the possibility of failure to relieve symptoms, and the possibility of symptom recurrence. A patient's specific risk factors, comorbidities, and intervention approach should be considered when discussing their prognosis. Before undergoing surgery, it is important to consider the potential complications and risks of the operation. Nevertheless, even if symptoms persist or return postoperatively, some patients may still benefit from the surgery and, with limited treatment options, may be worth trying.

If symptoms do persist or recur after 6 months, patients should undergo repeat testing including mesenteric duplex ultrasound, CTA/MRA, and celiac plexus block to evaluate for recurrence and help inform the decision for or against a revision operation. If a revision operation is considered, a conversation with the patient is crucial regarding increased risks, complications, and overall poorer prognosis when compared to a primary operation. With revision operations, there is a higher likelihood of adhesions and less ability to delineate anatomy, as well as a greater risk of arterial injury. A team approach is recommended including foregut and vascular surgery; if a foregut surgeon is primarily performing the revision operation, they should be in close contact with a vascular surgeon who can assist should an immediate need arise.

Conclusion

Surgical intervention is considered the mainstay of treatment for MALS and generally leads to symptom relief and improved quality of life. Additional follow-up data is needed to better define long-term outcomes, counsel patients with realistic expectations, determine if a revision operation is indicated and its potential outcomes, as well as describe other adjunctive interventions to help with long-term improvements in quality of life, if necessary. From the current limited data, there is about a 50% chance of patients experiencing some MALS symptom improvement after a revision operation. Further research is needed from other disciplines, such as gastroenterology, neurology, and rheumatology, among other specialties, to optimize long-term management for patients with this complex condition. Collaborative decision-making between the patient, surgeon, and others on their care team is necessary for the best treatment choices to be made for the patient.

References

1. Jimenez JC, Harlander-Locke M, Dutson EP. Open and laparoscopic treatment of median arcuate ligament syndrome. J Vasc Surg. 2012;56(3):869–73. https://doi.org/10.1016/j.jvs.2012.04.057.
2. Baccari P, Civilini E, Dordoni L, Melissano G, Nicoletti R, Chiesa R. Celiac artery compression syndrome managed by laparoscopy. J Vasc Surg. 2009;50(1):134–9. https://doi.org/10.1016/j.jvs.2008.11.124.
3. Roseborough GS. Laparoscopic management of celiac artery compression syndrome. J Vasc Surg. 2009;50(1):124–33. https://doi.org/10.1016/j.jvs.2008.12.078.
4. Kazmi SSH, Safi N, Berge ST, Kazmi M, Sundhagen JO, Hisdal J. Laparoscopic surgery for median arcuate ligament syndrome (MALS): a prospective cohort of 52 patients. Vasc Health Risk Manag. 2022;18:139–51. https://doi.org/10.2147/VHRM.S350841.
5. Metz FM, Blauw JTM, Brusse-Keizer M, Kolkman JJ, Bruno MJ, Geelkerken RH. Systematic review of the efficacy of treatment for median arcuate ligament syndrome. Eur J Vasc Endovasc Surg. 2022;64(6):720–32. https://doi.org/10.1016/j.ejvs.2022.08.033.
6. Pather K, Kärkkäinen JM, Tenorio ER, et al. Long-term symptom improvement and health-related quality of life after operative management of median arcuate ligament syndrome. J Vasc Surg. 2021;73(6):2050–8.e4. https://doi.org/10.1016/J.JVS.2020.10.074.
7. DeCicco J, Raja F, Ganesan S, El-Hayek K. First description of a histopathologic grading system and relationship to outcomes after robotic median arcuate ligament release with celiac ganglionectomy and lymphadenectomy. Surgery. 2024;175(3):822–32. https://doi.org/10.1016/J.SURG.2023.09.024.
8. Kam K, Ho F, Walker P, et al. Outcome predictors in median arcuate ligament syndrome. J Vasc Surg. 2017;65:1745–52. https://doi.org/10.1016/j.jvs.2016.11.040.
9. Birkhold M, Khalifeh A, Nagarsheth K, Kavic SM. Median arcuate ligament syndrome is effectively relieved with minimally invasive surgery. JSLS : Journal of the Society of Laparoscopic & Robotic Surgeons. 2022;26:4. https://doi.org/10.4293/JSLS.2022.00067.
10. Reilly LM, Ammar AD, Stoney RJ, Ehrenfeld WK. Late results following operative repair for celiac artery compression syndrome. J Vasc Surg. 1985;2(1):79–91. https://doi.org/10.1016/0741-5214(85)90177-6.
11. Morales-Soto W, Gonzales J, Jackson WF, Gulbransen BD. Enteric glia promote visceral hypersensitivity during inflammation through intercellular signaling with gut nociceptors. Sci Signal. 2023;16:812. https://doi.org/10.1126/SCISIGNAL.ADG1668.
12. Le Berre C, Naveilhan P, Rolli-Derkinderen M. Enteric glia at center stage of inflammatory bowel disease. Neurosci Lett. 2023:809. https://doi.org/10.1016/j.neulet.2023.137315.
13. Scavuzzo MA, Letai KC, Maeno-Hikichi Y, et al. Enteric glial hub cells coordinate intestinal motility. bioRxiv . Published online June. 2023;9 https://doi.org/10.1101/2023.06.07.544052.
14. Scavuzzo M. The way you move. Science (1979). 2023;382(6670):527–8. https://doi.org/10.1126/SCIENCE.ADK3883/ASSET/B56A5F0D-9ED8-4838-A512-79715CF8A4BF/ASSETS/IMAGES/LARGE/SCIENCE.ADK3883-F5.JPG.
15. Klimas A, Lemmer A, Bergert H, Brodhun M, Scholbach T, Großer K. Laparoscopic treatment of celiac artery compression syndrome in children and adolescents. Vasa. 2015;44(4):305–12. https://doi.org/10.1024/0301-1526/A000446.

16. Skelly CL, Stiles-Shields C, Mak GZ, et al. The impact of psychiatric comorbidities on patient-reported surgical outcomes in adults treated for the median arcuate ligament syndrome. J Vasc Surg. 2018;68(5):1414–21. https://doi.org/10.1016/j.jvs.2017.12.078.
17. Brody F, Randall JA, Amdur RL, Sidawy AN. A predictive model for patients with median arcuate ligament syndrome. Surg Endosc. 2018;32(12):4860–6. https://doi.org/10.1007/S00464-018-6240-Y/TABLES/4.
18. Cienfuegos JA, Estevez MG, Ruiz-Canela M, et al. Laparoscopic treatment of median arcuate ligament syndrome: analysis of long-term outcomes and predictive factors. J Gastrointest Surg. 2018;22(4):713–21. https://doi.org/10.1007/S11605-017-3635-3/METRICS.
19. Columbo JA, Trus T, Nolan B, et al. Contemporary management of median arcuate ligament syndrome provides early symptom improvement. J Vasc Surg. 2015;62(1):151–6. https://doi.org/10.1016/J.JVS.2015.01.050.
20. Rose SJ, Hartnett J, Madris B, Hsu R. Evaluation of a pain management program for patients with median arcuate ligament syndrome. SAGE Open Med. 2023:11. https://doi.org/10.1177/20503121231176636/SUPPL_FILE/SJ-DOCX-2-SMO-10.1177_20503121231176636.DOCX.
21. Do MV, Smith TA, Bazan HA, Sternbergh WC, Abbas AE, Richardson WS. Laparoscopic versus robot-assisted surgery for median arcuate ligament syndrome. Surg Endosc. 2013;27(11):4060–6. https://doi.org/10.1007/S00464-013-3061-X/TABLES/4.
22. Weber JM, Boules M, Fong K, et al. Median arcuate ligament syndrome is not a vascular disease. Ann Vasc Surg. 2016;30:22–7. https://doi.org/10.1016/j.avsg.2015.07.013.
23. Stiles-Shields C, Osos S, Heilbrun A, et al. Targeting coping to improve surgical outcomes in pediatric patients with median arcuate ligament syndrome: feasibility study. Front Psychol. 2021:12. https://doi.org/10.3389/FPSYG.2021.695435.
24. Strong A, Fong KE, Abraham B, Rodriguez JH, Park WM, Kroh MD. Reoperative laparoscopic release of median arcuate ligament. J Am Coll Surg. 2017;225(4):S221. https://doi.org/10.1016/J.JAMCOLLSURG.2017.07.512.
25. Edimo CO, Wajsberg JR, Wong S, Nahmias ZP, Riley BA. The dermatological aspects of hEDS in women. Int J Womens Dermatol. 2021;7(3):285. https://doi.org/10.1016/J.IJWD.2021.01.020.
26. Stembridge N, Doolan BJ, Lavallee ME, et al. The role of cutaneous manifestations in the diagnosis of the Ehlers-Danlos syndromes. Skin Health Dis. 2023;3(1):e140. https://doi.org/10.1002/SKI2.140.
27. A hypertrophic scar in a patient with hypermobility type, Ehlers–Danlos syndrome. J Am Acad Dermatol. 2017;76(6):AB15. https://doi.org/10.1016/J.JAAD.2017.04.077.
28. El-Hayek KM, Titus J, Bui A, Mastracci T, Kroh M. Laparoscopic median arcuate ligament release: are we improving symptoms? J Am Coll Surg. 2013;216:272–9. https://doi.org/10.1016/j.jamcollsurg.2012.10.004.

Chapter 18
The Median Arcuate Ligament Syndrome Journey: A Patient Perspective

Robin Insley Schrader, Suzanne Keppley Peek, Laura Gilmore, Tanya M. Holton, and Diane Gilmore

Pre-Diagnosis

Deciding to Seek Help

MALS patients often feel as though their bodies have betrayed them. Initial symptoms might present in a manner that most write off as nothing serious. Minor stomachache, difficulty running, or struggling to catch a breath going up the stairs are minor symptoms that might continue for years before patients seek professional care. Patients need medical providers who are willing to listen to their full history and who are dedicated to helping them find the answers to their symptoms with a proper diagnosis and treatment plan. For some patients, this might be a short process, but for many, a MALS diagnosis is a journey that takes years of self-advocacy and perseverance in the face of symptoms that do not clearly indicate the necessity of a clinical diagnosis.

Struggle of the Diagnostic Process

The challenge of connecting all the dots related to symptomology and receiving the correct diagnosis and treatment plan is difficult due to perceptions that MALS is exceedingly rare or not an actual diagnosis. Patients might be told they do not fit the perception of standard parameters for weight, age, or gender that might indicate a MALS diagnosis and leave appointments without answers. This lack of support often leaves patients feeling demoralized and hopeless.

R. I. Schrader · S. K. Peek (✉) · L. Gilmore · T. M. Holton · D. Gilmore
National MALS Foundation, Dedham, MA, USA
e-mail: robin@malsfoundation.org

D. Shouhed et al. (eds.), *Median Arcuate Ligament Syndrome*,
https://doi.org/10.1007/978-3-031-80740-4_18

Patients often have appointments with multiple specialists who conduct various tests that frequently appear "normal." When symptoms remain unresolved or worsen and diagnostic criteria are variable between providers, patients sometimes need to locate a different provider in order to secure appropriate testing and an accurate diagnosis. The years of continued searching and testing coupled with a diminishing quality of life exact an unquantifiable mental, emotional, and physical toll on both the patient and their caregivers until a diagnosis is finally made and treatment begins.

Recognizing the Burden Experienced by Patients and Caregivers

MALS patients and caregivers often learn strong advocacy skills, and sometimes this can present as frustration, strong opinions, hopelessness, and fear. The cycle of appointments and testing without answers frequently results in patients and caregivers feeling defeated, so they begin looking to support groups and online sites for answers. Engagement on social media platforms typically includes the patient journey, education, and research, even as this can sometimes lead to misinformation as well. Patients and caregivers often feel more empowered and hopeful through the knowledge they gain, which can enable further communication with their doctors. Research through both Internet and social media resources is not a replacement for clinical advice, but it can help patients and caregivers find the right doctors or facilities with the necessary experience for a MALS diagnosis. Finding the right provider for a particular MALS presentation is often the most challenging part of the MALS Journey.

Patients often try to hide the worst of their challenges from those around them. This can include their caregivers as they want to avoid becoming a burden. Caregivers can also struggle emotionally during the diagnostic process as they can feel helpless in watching their loved one suffer debilitating symptoms. Having support for caregivers as well as the patient is essential. Caregivers play a significant role in ensuring that patients do not feel isolated and have someone to support them through their journey. Thus, it is important that they also are included in clinical discussions so that they too do not feel isolated.

Diagnosis and Surgery

Relief of Diagnosis

Being an undiagnosed patient is profoundly isolating. Not having an official diagnosis makes it harder to explain symptoms to caregivers, educators, coworkers, managers, and other people in the patient's life. This can result in feelings of isolation, depression, anxiety, and physical depletion. Ironically, a diagnosis often provides a much-needed morale boost to the patient. In addition to relief, they might also feel fear when receiving their diagnosis as their journey to feeling better has just begun and the prospect of surgery can seem overwhelming.

Reality of Finding Treatment

Once MALS is diagnosed, finding a doctor to pursue treatment is the next challenge for the patient. Many patients consult multiple surgeons and often feel as though there are conflicting opinions on treatment. Due to the history of diagnostic struggle, conflicting clinical opinions can often leave the patient feeling unsure of how to proceed. Having a provider who recognizes this struggle and reassures the patient with clinically accurate, factual information can be reassuring and can help feel as though there is a partnership between the doctor and the patient. It is this partnership that moves MALS patients closer to better health, healing, and well-being.

Choosing the Right Operative Treatment

The National MALS Foundation works hard to combat misinformation in the patient community regarding surgical approaches. The choice between open, laparoscopic, or robotic surgery is often confusing for the patient in light of misinformation online, challenges with finances, and fear about not having positive outcomes. Patients feel uncertain about which approach is optimal for them and benefit from having open and honest conversations about all the different surgical approaches.

Importance of Managing Patient Expectations Prior to Surgery

Prior to surgery, patients appreciate having discussions regarding expectations for recovery and management of symptoms. Helping patients understand the differences between surgical healing time and the time it takes their bodies to feel the full benefits from surgery is critical in postoperative outcomes. Discussions about defining a successful surgery are also beneficial as often this might be different for the surgeon and the patient. Patients and their caregivers struggle with the reality that MALS symptom resolution can vary due to individual circumstances. Clear communication between the doctor and patient/caregiver about these expectations can help alleviate postoperative stress and improve recovery.

Patients often report surgical pain resolving within 6–8 weeks, depending on the approach; however, symptom improvement often takes longer. Sometimes, patients report symptoms worsening within the first few months of surgery. Many patients report symptom improvement starting after surgical healing and many indicate they do not feel the full benefit of surgery for 6–12 months or longer. These timelines are important to know prior to surgery. Otherwise, patients can feel as though surgery is unsuccessful when, in reality, there simply has not been enough recovery time.

Patients also benefit from discussing potential options should surgery not provide the outcome they hoped. If symptoms do recur, patients often think it is due to failed surgical intervention when instead it may be caused by common postoperative conditions that doctors can prepare patients for during presurgery consultations. Patients also benefit from discussing potential options should surgery not provide the outcome they hoped. Patients feel supported in postoperative symptoms management when short- and long-term follow-up is provided.

Preparing for Hospitalization and Surgery

In addition to managing the symptoms of MALS while preparing for surgery, patients report that it is essential to have information about how to prepare to go to the hospital, what to expect during their hospital stay, and how to prepare adequately for life at home following surgery. Being informed allows the patient to focus on healing and can help reduce the stress that surrounds surgery.

Here are some items MALS patients find comforting and helpful:

- Small pillow to press against the belly/incision.
- Blanket from home.
- Dry shampoo.
- Lotion for hands or face to help with dry skin.
- Long phone or iPad charger.
- Earplugs.
- Hair ties.

Surgery

Patients often need clarification about the basics of surgery. The patient community is full of misinformation and personal prejudices, which can lead to patients being unsure of what is being done during their procedure. Being clear and concise with patients about what surgery looks like is helpful.

Waking up from any surgery can be scary for patients. Discussing realistic expectations with the patient prior to surgery is helpful to prevent anxiety and patients benefit from knowing the different aspects of the surgical process, length of hospitalization, post-op pain management while hospitalized, and discharge planning.

Discharge

Patients report being sent home too quickly or with inadequate instructions for symptom management, and this can often result in ER visits. In addition, patients need to be prepared for how surgery might impact their travel home. Discussing what typical issues might arise while traveling can help ease the patient's mind.

Home Recovery

Preparing the patient and caregiver for the return home is an integral part of patient recovery. Clinicians can help by advising patients and caregivers about how surgery might limit both short- and long-term activities like driving, housework, cooking, eating, exercising, and returning to work or school. Doctors can help set the tone that healing is lengthy and that patients and caregivers need to be compassionate with themselves.

Postoperative patients frequently report difficulty with dysregulated eating and postoperative nausea. Preparing for these concerns and having a plan to support them help reassure patients during their recovery at home.

The recovery process itself can strain relationships. Not every MALS patient has adequate support at home, and even if they do, patients find online support groups vital during this time. Online groups can relieve isolation and help people connect with others who understand the MALS journey. Surgeons can help by sharing successful patient stories, connecting patients with other patients, and encouraging the patient to seek out online support groups.

Psychosocial Impact of MALS

MALS can impact a person's mental health, especially if left untreated long after symptoms begin. Isolation can form and contribute to loneliness, depression, anxiety, and poor coping skills. Relationships with partners or family members might change, and friendships might start to fade as patients sink further into life with illness. This can leave patients feeling like there is nowhere to turn.

It is essential to recognize how illness impacts the patient's cognitive, social, emotional, mental, and behavioral health. MALS and its impacts can be isolating. Many recommendations for positive mental health focus on healthy eating, engaging in social activities, and exercising regularly, but these suggestions are often difficult for patients with MALS. It is essential to help the patient understand that all patients with MALS are different and that finding activities and support to reduce stress levels, cope with isolation, and take care of their mind, body, and soul is an individual process of trial and error. When referring patients to counseling support to help with surgical expectations, post-op outcomes, and symptom management, it is critical to validate the patient's real physical symptoms associated with the clinical condition itself. Otherwise, patients might interpret a counseling referral as a dismissal of symptoms and feel unheard.

Role of Patient Advocacy and Online Community Support

Online Support Groups

An online support group is immensely beneficial to both patients and caregivers. These groups are a safe place for patients to discuss their struggles and their MALS Journey. They allow patients to vent, ask questions, and seek support from those who understand what they are going through. These groups provide a sense of community, help patients know they are not alone, and provide ideas for activities, coping strategies, symptom management, etc. Patients and caregivers often build meaningful relationships with people worldwide experiencing a similar health journey. This can ease the emotional burden many patients experience.

Patient Advocacy

Advocates come in many forms: parents, friends, professionals, or foundations. The National MALS Foundation advocates on behalf of the MALS community. The Foundation helps to educate the MALS community with accurate information that can help them on the path to receiving answers. The Foundation also provides scientifically grounded information to doctors looking for answers for their patients.

Patient advocacy highlights the need for the patient's voice to be heard within the medical community to encourage doctor-patient collaboration and trust. By spreading MALS awareness in the medical community, the National MALS Foundation hopes to reduce delay times in getting a diagnosis and expedite the implementation of the best treatment plan for the patient. The Foundation strives to make visible the invisible as a meaningful way to show support and advocate for patients' health and well-being.

The Foundation also advocates for collaboration within the medical community. A core tenet in medicine is education, the art of discovery, and sharing that wealth of information with others. The MALS Foundation advocates for additional research, establishing standardized protocols, and standardizing the surgical process. Having doctors do the same is essential for helping MALS patients.

Conclusion

The journey of a patient with MALS is a marathon, not a sprint. Doctors play an essential role in helping patients through the diagnostic, surgical, and postoperative phases of care. Ensuring that patients are given realistic expectations about things like postoperative complications, timelines for surgical recovery, and the time it can take a patient to feel the full benefits of surgery is essential. Above all, patients value doctors who understand that they are not looking for a provider with all the answers, but one with the patience, empathy, and willingness to help them find answers and improve their daily life. The National MALS Foundation plays an important role in bringing together the community of MALS clinicians as well as patients and families to improve clinical knowledge and the patient experience.

Index

D. Shouhed et al. (eds.), *Median Arcuate Ligament Syndrome*,
https://doi.org/10.1007/978-3-031-80740-4

MIX
Papier aus verantwortungsvollen Quellen
Paper from responsible sources
FSC® C105338

If you have any concerns about our products,
you can contact us on
ProductSafety@springernature.com

In case Publisher is established outside the EU,
the EU authorized representative is:
Springer Nature Customer Service Center GmbH
Europaplatz 3, 69115 Heidelberg, Germany

Printed by Libri Plureos GmbH
in Hamburg, Germany